AF705282

"Renn offers something rare: a genuinely integrative account that bridges theory, research and the realities of therapeutic work. The book shows a sophisticated grasp of developmental and relational processes while remaining clinically alive and deeply attuned to human vulnerability. Conceptually ambitious and practically useful, it will be indispensable for clinicians, trainees and scholars."

Professor Peter Fonagy, *Head of Division, Psychology & Language Sciences, UCL, National Clinical Adviser for Children's Mental Health, NHSE*

"This book is a gem. Renn skilfully bridges diverse ways of understanding and practising psychotherapy. He links mind and body, relational and traditional psychotherapy, attachment, neurobiology and the consulting room, the intrapsychic and sociopolitical, the past, present and future. He explains complex ideas with clarity and shows how they can be integrated. Renn gets to the heart of the curative processes in psychotherapy and offers hope for healing rifts in the field."

Dr. Graham Music, *Consultant Psychotherapist, Tavistock Centre, Trainer and Author*

"Renn provides a masterly integration of diverse perspectives on understanding and treating cumulative trauma, with attention to lifespan and intergenerational impacts. His volume will benefit novice and senior clinicians seeking a contemporary psychoanalytic, neuroscientific and attachment-oriented account. Rarely have Bowlby and Klein appeared together with such appreciation for each. His clinical vignettes show how a relational-neurodevelopmental framework can transform this nuanced form of trauma through meaningful relational encounters."

Howard Steele, *Professor of Psychology, The New School, New York City, and Editor, Attachment & Human Development*

Relational Foundations

This book develops a relational-neurodevelopmental framework for understanding how early experience becomes procedurally encoded, organised, and transmitted across generations.

Drawing on three decades of clinical practice, it brings psychoanalysis, attachment theory, infant observation, and neuroscience into close dialogue with the lived moment of therapeutic work. At its centre is the concept of cumulative relational trauma, offering a way to understand developmental harm as emerging through ongoing relational processes rather than discrete events. Structured in four parts, the volume addresses key clinical domains, including enactment, sexuality, power, forensic settings, and psychosis, while remaining grounded in practice. It shows how change unfolds through sustained relational engagement, affect regulation, and reparative processes over time.

Written for psychotherapists, clinicians, and scholars, this book offers an integrative, ethically attuned account of development that honours complexity.

Paul Renn is a UKCP-accredited psychoanalytic psychotherapist, supervisor, and couples therapist in London. He has a background in the National Probation Service and is on the editorial board of *Psychoanalytic Inquiry*. He has published widely and is the author of *The Silent Past and the Invisible Present* (Routledge, 2012).

Relational Foundations

A Relational-Neurodevelopmental Approach to Cumulative Trauma in Clinical Practice

Paul Renn

Routledge
Taylor & Francis Group
LONDON AND NEW YORK

Designed cover image: Getty Images

First published 2027
by Routledge
4 Park Square, Milton Park, Abingdon, Oxon OX14 4RN

and by Routledge
605 Third Avenue, New York, NY 10158

Routledge is an imprint of the Taylor & Francis Group, an informa business

© 2027 Paul Renn

The right of Paul Renn to be identified as author of this work has been asserted in accordance with sections 77 and 78 of the Copyright, Designs and Patents Act 1988.

All rights reserved. No part of this book may be reprinted or reproduced or utilised in any form or by any electronic, mechanical, or other means, now known or hereafter invented, including photocopying and recording, or in any information storage or retrieval system, without permission in writing from the publishers.

Trademark notice: Product or corporate names may be trademarks or registered trademarks, and are used only for identification and explanation without intent to infringe.

For Product Safety Concerns and Information please contact our EU representative GPSR@taylorandfrancis.com. Taylor & Francis Verlag GmbH, Kaufingerstraße 24, 80331 München, Germany.

British Library Cataloguing in Publication Data
A catalogue record for this book is available from the British Library

ISBN: 9781041338161 (hbk)
ISBN: 9781041334781 (pbk)
ISBN: 9781003789727 (ebk)

DOI: 10.4324/9781003789727

Typeset in Optima
by Taylor & Francis Books

To my children, Nic and Claire, their partners, Nicci and Tom, and my granddaughter, Rosa

Contents

About the Author

Paul Renn is a UKCP-accredited psychoanalytic psychotherapist, training therapist, supervisor, and couples therapist in private practice in London. He trained at the Centre for Attachment-based Psychoanalytic Psychotherapy (now the Bowlby Centre) and has a professional background in the National Probation Service, where he specialised in work with violent individuals and couples. He is a member of the International Association for Forensic Psychotherapy and the International Association for Relational Psychoanalysis and Psychotherapy, and serves on the editorial board of *Psychoanalytic Inquiry*, for which he also edited a special issue on the creative role of attachment theory in clinical practice. He is the author of *The Silent Past and the Invisible Present: Memory, Trauma, and Representation in Psychotherapy* (Routledge, 2012). He has published widely in journals and has presented CPD workshops and seminars in the UK and internationally.

Foreword

This is a book for practising psychotherapists. Readers are reminded that our author's first role was as a professional oboist. No surprise then that throughout this delightful yet research-grounded text Renn demonstrates perfect pitch for the music of psychotherapy sessions – their melodies, harmonies, key changes, discords, resolutions, development, and closing cadences, perfect and imperfect.

Based on a lifetime of psychotherapeutic thinking, reading and practice, Renn's project is to explore and synthesise the disparate theoretical foundations of attachment-informed relational psychoanalytic psychotherapy. While it may seem tautologous to quote from a volume upon which the reader is about to embark, this passage encapsulates the essence of Renn's theoretical viewpoint. I have highlighted some of the key concepts he addresses:

> this volume … traces the *developmental architecture of internal worlds*, the role of early caregiving in shaping *affective regulation*, and the intergenerational transmission of *unprocessed emotional states* … Persecutory anxieties … can [be] understood as the psychic residue of *cumulative relational trauma* – chronic emotional inconsistency, parental anxiety and depression, unspoken conflict, and repeated *disruptions to the child's sense of safety*.

The aim of this foreword is to give readers a taster of a number of these themes. The central thread running throughout the book is that of cumulative relational trauma (CRT). The notion of CRT is inherently normative. It contrasts with healthy developmental care-seeker/caregiver experiences characterised by empathy, mentalising, turn-taking, affect co-regulation, playfulness, rupture-repair cycles, and respect for privacy and autonomy. CRT builds on and is consistent with Herman's (1992) notion of complex trauma, van der Kolk's (1994) "body keeps the score" psychosomatism, and Main's model of disorganised attachment (Fonagy, 1998). The CRT model extends the conventional understanding of the term trauma which typically implies a penetrative (the term's etymology derives from "to pierce"), unanticipated, damaging event such as a sudden bereavement, illness or accident, or single acts of perverse exploitation such as physical or sexual abuse.

Thus, from a CRT perspective, rather than malign presence or intrusion, one of the most damaging adverse childhood experiences is neglect, traumatic by the very absence of a loving relational field. The developmental relational perspective also shifts the perspective on trauma away from a unidirectional perpetrator-victim model to a relational one. Psychopathology derives from children's attempts to achieve a modicum of security in the context in which they find themselves, however developmentally maladaptive that may be. A telling illustration of this is the finding that girls classified as disorganised in the strange situation aged 1–1½ reach menarche on average 10 months earlier than their securely attached counterparts. This finding shows that attachment dispositions have physiological underpinnings, and that what is conventionally viewed as diagnostic psychopathology can be more usefully seen as adaptation to adversity (Ellis, 2004). If a child's environment is disorganised and unpredictable, there are good evolutionary reasons for reaching sexual maturity early in order to ensure genetic survival into the next generation. Similarly, if care-giving is perfunctory or roughly administered, then self-sufficiency or seemingly "masochistic" strategies will be needed in order to maintain a degree of relational security.

While these psycho-physiological processes go on entirely below consciousness, and are inherently beyond the individual's control, they have profound interpersonal implications, and form the core of psychotherapeutic work. As Renn convincingly demonstrates, in seeking help, these pre- or non-verbal procedural expectations and relational patterns will be brought into the consulting room and played out transferentially. The role of the therapist is (a) to identify these patterns in her own mind, (b) to find ways to encourage the client to self-mentalise so that they begin to reach conscious awareness, (c) to reduce the shame and guilt associated with psychological illness by seeing their self-defeating patterns as adaptive, and (d) to begin to create a consulting room culture in which control and/or chaos are replaced by care and communication.

A degree of trauma is inherent in the human condition. Which of us has not suffered a degree of loss, failure, illness or oppression? But in non-pathological situations the impact of these slings and arrows of outrageous fortune are mitigated by affect co-regulation with the help of a caring other, or in Bowlby's term, a secure base. The second key concept in the relational perspective therefore is that of affect regulation. Relational trauma has two components. There is the trauma itself – neglect, insensitivity, caregiver depression or paranoia, absence, prolonged and repeated abuse. Concomitant with this, CRT implies the absence of, or interference with, the holding, containing and soothing which a secure base figure can offer to the traumatised child. Failures of parenting are universal; indeed, in Winnicott's model it is the job of parents to fail, providing the child with first steps towards independence of mind and agency. But in good-enough parent child relationships the caregiver recognises the child's distress and helps them to repair the everyday ruptures that are the stuff of family life. Anxiety is soothed; depression alleviated; persecutory fears defanged.

In CRT these processes are absent, disavowed, or distorted. Based on their own traumatic developmental histories, caregivers may fail to recognise the child's distress, override, dismiss, exploit or invalidate it. In the relational model which Renn advocates, affect regulation becomes the central plank of therapeutic work, especially in relation to the range of negative affects which clients bring to therapy – misery, depression, shame, self-loathing, feelings of inadequacy or destructiveness. Attachment research shows that insecurely attached parents find it especially difficult to accept and regulate their children's expressions of negative feelings – "meltdowns" as they are these days termed (Kim et al., 2014). Therapy cannot change the past. What it can do is offer an experience of affect regulation previously unavailable to the client. Renn's clinical examples beautifully illustrate the process of "staying with" the client's bad feelings – not brushing them aside or hastily trying to alleviate them, but reformulating them in a wider context of survival, and using empathy and humour to help clients move on from their entrenched negativity. When things go well, over time, this becomes internalised and forms part of the sufferer's repertoire of self-soothing skills.

This brings us to the third component of Renn's relational perspective. CRT is procedural rather than primarily episodic. Isolated episodes of trauma in an otherwise health-yielding environment are usually recoverable. The therapist's job, rather than pinpointing "causal" traumatogenic moments, is to be sensitive to the relational patterns which clients set up in their own lives, often maladaptively, and specifically in the consulting room – although, that said, these patterns may be helpfully epitomised by a particular incident or anecdote.

There are important consequences of this viewpoint. First, therapist's conceptual models need to be complex and multifaceted rather than simplistic and linear. Field theory suggests that clients' difficulties be seen as the external emanations of intertwined subterranean threads of sociopolitical, genetic, and developmental processes. This presents a technical problem, in that therapeutic interventions work best as snappy, easily memorable interventions. Renn's answer here, I suspect, is that the therapists' primary tools are her own intuitive and emotional reactions to the client's actions and non-actions. This entails a therapeutic stance of "triple listening" (Holmes, 2024) – listening to the clients' stories (or absent stories), listening to oneself listening (i.e. "reading" one's countertransference), and listening to the way the client responds to one's responses, and, where necessary modifying one's words and the tone in which they are delivered in order to co-create a more attuned linguistic mutuality.

The fourth aspect of Renn's 4:4 time signature concerns the neuroscience underpinnings of psychotherapeutic work. He draws on Gallese's discovery of mirror neurones, and Schore's (1994) emphasis on right brain to right brain communication in the mother-infant relationship to argue that relational neuroscience underpins the psychotherapeutic perspectives he champions. To this I would add the work of Karl Friston and the free energy principle (Holmes, 2020; 2024). Friston (2010) shows mathematically how the brain/mind aims always to minimise the "free energy" or "surprisal" of incoming sensory information about the environment including the interpersonal environment. We cling to pre-existing "top-down" models of the world in ways that explain transference (seeing the present in the light of the past) and/or by attempting to seek out or shape the world in the light of prior expectations (i.e. "projective identification"). Friston and Frith's "a duet for one" model shows how, using the "borrowed brain" of a trusted intimate other (which can include a therapist), more accurate and adaptive models of the world can be generated (Friston & Frith, 2015).

This brings us, finally, to Renn's model of how psychotherapy brings about change. To quote him once more, his starting point is the ways in which "the silent relational past lives on in invisible ways in the interpersonal present". Renn's accounts of mutative moments in therapy rely on a number of simple yet profound ideas. These include the need through attunement to bring about "moments of meeting" where the free energy of surprise generates new meanings; helping the client to move towards "earned security" in place of disorganised or preoccupied patterns of attachment; the need for therapists to draw on their bodily feelings to identify implicit relational patterns which can then be verbalised; helping the client to reclaim disowned or dissociated aspects of the self's affective repertoire – anger, sadness, joy even; creating confrontations or addressing impasses in which the client's habitual methods of survival no longer apply, thus opening up a space in which new more adaptive relational patterns, including Stern's "vitality affects" can emerge; accepting the inevitability of transference/countertransference enactments co-created by therapist and client, and finding ways to highlight and mentalise these.

I end with two vivid examples of the ways in which Renn, secure in his theoretical foundations, allows himself to take risks. He courageously shows us how he walks a high wire between risk taking and enactment, in ways that vitalise and transform embedded dissociations and maladaptive patterns of relating. Here he is waiting for a response to an intervention that confounded the client's expectation of criticism or rejection: "I gazed back with bright eyes, smiled warmly, tilted my head to the left and, with a slightly quizzical, yet challenging, expression, raised my eyebrows and waited." And here, after a risky but emotionally rich response to a client's confession of erotic transference, he reveals himself communicating "a feisty struggle about boundaries, but also by emotional honesty, humour, playfulness, and irony."

Reader, you will learn a lot from this book, which is both scholarly and playful, securely grounded in theory, yet able to respond in the moment to the client's lived reality with spontaneity and sensitivity. Using his own journey as example, Renn invites us to immerse ourselves deeply in the theoretical bases of relational psychotherapy, and then, trusting theory as our secure base, to throw off its shackles, and to learn to play, improvise, listen, and intuit. Both we, and our clients, will benefit.

Jeremy Holmes

References

Ellis, B. (2004). Timing of pubertal maturation in girls: An integrated life history approach. *Psychological Bulletin*, 130(6), 920–958.

Fonagy, P. (1998). An attachment theory approach to treatment of the difficult patient. *Bulletin of the Menninger Clinic*, 62(2), 147–169.

Friston, K. (2010). The free-energy principle: a unified brain theory? *Nature Reviews Neuroscience*, 11(2), 127–138.

Friston, K. & Frith, C. (2015). A duet for one: consciousness, action and neuroplasticity. *Cortex*, 70, 1–22.

Gallese, V. (2001). The "shared manifold" hypothesis. *Journal of Consciousness Studies*, 8(5–7), 33–50.

Herman, J. (1992). *Trauma and recovery*. New York: Basic Books.

Holmes, J. (2020). *The brain has a mind of its own*. London: Confer Books.

Holmes, J. (2024). *The spirit of psychotherapy*. London: Karnac.

Kim, S., Fonagy, P., Allen, J., Martinez, S.. Iyengar, U. & Strathearn, L; (2014). Mothers who are securely attached in pregnancy show more attuned infant mirroring 7 months postpartum. *Infant Behavior and Development*, 37(4), 491–503.

Schore, A. N. (1994). *Affect regulation and the origin of the self: The neurobiology of emotional development*. Hillsdale, NJ: Lawrence Erlbaum.

Stern, D. N., Sander, L. W., Nahum, J. P., Harrison, A. M., Lyons-Ruth, K., Morgan, A. C., Bruschweiler-Stern, N. & Tronick, E. Z. (1998). Non-interpretive mechanisms in psychoanalytic therapy: The "something more" than interpretation. *International Journal of Psychoanalysis*, 79, 903–921.

van der Kolk, B. A. (1994). The body keeps the score. *Harvard Review of Psychiatry*, 1(5), 253–265.

Introduction

Over the past thirty years of clinical practice, I have returned repeatedly to a fundamental question: how do the earliest relationships we experience continue to shape us across a lifetime? This question is not merely theoretical. It arises daily in the consulting room – in silences and repetitions, in what cannot be said, in relational patterns that feel both urgent and impossibly old. It appears in the way a patient hesitates before speaking, in the particular texture of their distress, and in configurations of relating that feel simultaneously familiar and strange.

This book brings together three decades of clinical work and theoretical reflection on attachment, trauma, and the intergenerational transmission of relational experience. It represents not a linear progression, but an iterative deepening: a return to core questions as clinical understanding and theoretical frameworks have evolved. The chapters trace my intellectual journey from early engagement with attachment theory and infant observation, through sustained exploration of cumulative relational trauma and its transmission, to later integration with contemporary neuroscience and relational psychoanalysis.

The concept that unifies this work is cumulative relational trauma – the subtle, chronic disruptions that occur even within ostensibly "good enough" caregiving environments and that shape implicit relational patterns across generations. This volume provides the first comprehensive articulation of this concept. Unlike discrete traumatic events, cumulative trauma operates through repeated misattunements, failures of recognition, and absences of repair. It is encoded in procedural memory systems, transmitted through the quality of relational engagement, and often remains outside conscious awareness. Understanding cumulative trauma requires holding together psychoanalytic depth, attachment research, developmental observation, and neuroscience, without reducing one perspective to another.

The Evolution of a Relational-Neurodevelopmental Framework

My early clinical training emphasised intrapsychic conflict and phantasy. While this lens offered valuable insights, it proved insufficient to account for

DOI: 10.4324/9781003789727-1

the powerful yet often wordless dimensions of clinical work that I encountered. Attachment theory provided a bridge, situating internal worlds within the matrix of lived relationships. Infant observation, undertaken during training, offered a visceral understanding of how patterns of attunement and misattunement become encoded in gesture, timing, and bodily regulation long before language emerges.

Work in forensic settings further sharpened my attention to trauma – not only the dramatic ruptures of abuse and violence, but the quieter, cumulative failures of containment and recognition that compromise the developing self. Increasingly, my clinical focus turned to how such patterns are transmitted across generations, how they emerge within the therapeutic relationship, and how transformation becomes possible through sustained relational engagement.

Integration with neuroscience came later, prompted by both opportunity and necessity. Research on affect regulation, implicit memory, and the neurobiology of attachment provided a somatic grounding for the clinical observations I had long made. At the same time, I remained cautious about biological reductionism. The challenge has been to hold neuroscience in dialogue with psychoanalytic and relational understanding – allowing each to inform the other without collapsing complexity into mechanism.

What has gradually emerged from this clinical and theoretical evolution is what I now describe as a *relational-neurodevelopmental framework*: an integrative orientation for understanding how mind, brain, and relational life co-evolve across development.

This framework proceeds from the understanding that the human brain is not an isolated, intrapsychic organ but a profoundly social one, shaped within relationships from the earliest moments of life. Neurodevelopment unfolds through processes of interpersonal regulation, affective exchange, and meaning-making, as caregivers – and later relational partners – participate in the calibration of arousal, the organisation of emotion, and the formation of internal worlds. Through neural plasticity and embodied memory, these relational experiences become instantiated in characteristic ways of feeling, perceiving, imagining, and relating.

Drawing together relational psychoanalysis, attachment theory, developmental psychology, and contemporary neuroscience, the framework situates neurobiological processes within lived relational contexts. Development is understood as dynamic and recursive rather than linear or predetermined, and open to transformation across the lifespan. Within this perspective, cumulative trauma can be understood as relationally patterned experience that becomes embodied, transmitted, and potentially revised through new relational encounters, including the therapeutic relationship.

The relational–neurodevelopmental framework is not a mechanistic model but a generative orientation – one that invites clinicians and theorists to think developmentally, relationally, and neurobiologically at once. The chapters that follow elaborate and extend this framework across developmental, clinical, and intergenerational domains.

Structure and Organisation of the Volume

The book is organised into four parts, each introduced by a brief orienting essay that situates the chapters within the book's overall developmental and clinical argument.

Part I ("Origins: Attachment, Development, and the Inner World") establishes the developmental foundations, examining how early attachment relationships shape the internal world and how implicit relational knowledge is formed through embodied interaction.

Part II ("Cumulative Trauma, Memory, and Intergenerational Transmission") develops cumulative trauma as the book's central organising concept, exploring how relational failures become encoded in memory and transmitted across generations.

Part III ("Relational Process and the Clinical Encounter") moves into the consulting room, examining how cumulative trauma is enacted within therapeutic relationships and how procedural transformation becomes possible through relational engagement.

Part IV ("Integration and Future Directions") brings these strands together, unfolding across four chapters. Together, these synthesise theory, clinical process, and neuroscience into a relational-neurodevelopmental framework, while opening towards future directions for practice and training.

Each orienting essay is intended to support continuity and integration, guiding the reader through the book's conceptual progression while allowing individual chapters to stand on their own.

Method, Voice, and Audience

Some chapters appear substantially as originally written, while others have been revised and integrated. This reflects the book's nature as both a collected body of work and an evolving argument. Where appropriate, retrospective reflections have been added to situate earlier writing within contemporary clinical and theoretical contexts.

Variation in chapter length reflects conceptual weight rather than editorial inconsistency. The extended treatment of cumulative relational trauma reflects its central role in the framework, while detailed clinical material is included because procedural knowledge resists summary – it emerges in the fine texture of relational process.

This book is written primarily for practicing psychoanalysts, psychotherapists, and mental health professionals working with attachment, trauma, and intergenerational processes. It assumes familiarity with psychoanalytic ideas while remaining accessible to readers from adjacent traditions. A glossary is provided to support navigation across theoretical languages.

Closing Reflections

Clinical work teaches humility about what we know and how we know it. Theory offers frameworks for thinking, but it cannot substitute for the lived, embodied reality of therapeutic encounter. Over time, my clinical experience has reinforced a simple but demanding insight: transformation occurs not through insight alone, but through relationship – through being encountered, recognised, and engaged with differently over time.

The patients whose experiences inform this volume have been my greatest teachers. Their willingness to risk vulnerability, to return after rupture, and to remain in relationship under difficult conditions has shaped both my thinking and my practice. I offer this book not as a set of answers, but as a contribution to an ongoing conversation about how experience becomes embodied, transmitted across generations, and revised through new relational encounters.

Part I

Origins: Attachment, Development, and the Inner World

Introduction to Part I

How do we become who we are? This enduring question takes on particular urgency when we consider the earliest relationships that shape the developing self. Part I establishes the developmental and theoretical foundations for understanding how attachment relationships give rise to the internal world, how patterns of security and insecurity emerge, and how early experience becomes encoded in implicit, procedural forms that persist across the lifespan.

The three chapters in this section examine the relational foundations of subjectivity – the processes through which interaction becomes internalisation, and relationship becomes self.

Chapter 1 sets out an integrative framework that brings classical psychoanalytic models of the internal world into dialogue with contemporary relational-developmental, attachment, and neurobiological perspectives. It challenges the opposition between intrapsychic and interpersonal, phantasy and reality, arguing instead for a both/and position in which internal worlds emerge through lived interaction, affective meaning, and embodied regulation. This epistemological stance – holding complexity without reduction – guides the entire volume.

Chapter 2 traces the developmental unfolding of attachment, security, separation, and differentiation. Drawing on psychoanalytic theory, empirical attachment research, and affective neuroscience, it shows how early relational experience shapes the capacity to explore, to separate, and to maintain connection across distance. Failures of containment and recognition are shown to compromise agency and to lay the groundwork for later cumulative trauma, introducing concepts – particularly misattunement and failures of repair – that become central in Part II.

Chapter 3 focuses on infant observation as both method and clinical resource. Infant observation provides access to the formation of implicit relational knowledge – the procedural patterns that emerge before language and persist as the procedural past. This chapter demonstrates how bodily

DOI: 10.4324/9781003789727-2

and affective processes encode patterns of attunement, misattunement, and repair, establishing a bridge between infancy research and adult psychotherapy. What appears later in the consulting room is not remembered experience but enacted knowing.

Taken together, these chapters establish that the internal world is relational in origin, formed through repeated interactions that become internalised regulatory patterns; that security depends not on the absence of rupture but on reliable repair; and that early experience is encoded primarily in implicit, procedural memory systems that shape relational engagement long before reflective thought or narrative is possible.

These propositions have direct clinical implications. If the internal world is formed through interaction, then transformation requires relational experience, not insight alone. If security rests on repair rather than perfection, then the therapeutic relationship becomes the site where new procedural patterns may emerge through cycles of rupture and reconnection. And if early experience operates implicitly, therapeutic work must engage enacted, embodied, and affective dimensions of relationship, not only explicit narrative and interpretation.

Part I therefore provides the developmental grounding for what follows. Understanding cumulative trauma (Part II) requires understanding how relational patterns are encoded; working therapeutically with these patterns (Part III) requires recognising their implicit, procedural nature; and integrating multiple perspectives; (Part IV) depends on a framework that holds developmental, psychoanalytic, and neurobiological perspectives in productive tension without reduction.

As you read these chapters, I invite you to keep in mind a central question that animates the entire volume: what does it mean that we are formed in relationship – not as pre-existing subjects who then relate, but as selves whose very organisation emerges through the quality of engagement we experience?

1 Towards an Integrative Psychoanalysis of the Internal World

Retrospective Reflection

As I look back across the decades that have shaped my clinical work, I am struck by how the field has continually moved towards what the consulting room has always revealed: that the internal world is not an isolated chamber of drives but a living, relational system. The theories that inform this volume did not arrive as abstract frameworks; they emerged in dialogue with patients whose struggles, resilience, and relational longings have been my most enduring teachers.

Over the years, I have found myself returning to the same questions with renewed depth: How does the past live in the body? How do early relational patterns become procedural truths that shape the self long before they can be spoken? And how, within the therapeutic relationship, do these patterns soften, reorganise, or transform? These questions have guided my engagement with psychoanalysis, attachment theory, developmental research, and contemporary neuroscience – not as competing traditions, but as complementary lenses through which to understand the lived experience of cumulative trauma. The concept of cumulative relational trauma introduced here is developed in depth in Chapter 5, where its mechanisms, clinical manifestations, and intergenerational transmission are examined in detail.

This opening chapter traces the intellectual and clinical journey that has informed my work. It is offered in the spirit of gratitude – to the thinkers who expanded the field, to the patients who deepened my understanding, and to the ongoing relational dialogue between them that continues to animate the consulting room. The pages that follow reflect this integrative stance: theoretically grounded, clinically humble, and rooted in the belief that the internal world remains open to transformation through relationship.

Introduction

The internal world is not a static archive of the past, it is a living, breathing relational system. For thirty years, my clinical practice has been a dialogue

DOI: 10.4324/9781003789727-3

between the profound depths of psychoanalytic theory and the lived reality of patients grappling with "cumulative trauma" – those subtle, persistent relational failures that occur even in "good enough" families. It is a world populated not just by biological drives but by the ghosts of early caregivers and the echoes of unremembered experiences. When we speak of the "internal world", we are describing the psychic landscape where the past meets the present and where the self is perpetually co-created in the presence of the other.

As the opening to this volume, this chapter seeks to do more than merely summarise the history of psychoanalytic thought. It aims to act as a guide for a specific way of working – one that is theoretically robust yet clinically humble. To understand how early relational experiences are encoded in the body and transmitted across generations we must first trace a specific intellectual trajectory. This journey represents a paradigmatic shift in psychoanalysis: a move away from seeing the mind as a closed system of drives and towards an integrative perspective that recognises the primacy of the relationship.

The chapters that follow are the fruit of three decades of engagement with these themes. They bridge the gap between classical theory and contemporary research, moving from the intrapsychic to the intersubjective. By re-examining the foundations of our field through the lens of attachment research and neuroscience, we can begin to see the internal world not as a fixed destination but as a dynamic process of relating that remains open to transformation within the therapeutic encounter.

The Intrapsychic Anchor: From Drive to Object

Classical psychoanalysis began by looking inwards, searching for the origins of human suffering within the biological impulses of the individual. Sigmund Freud's original topographic and structural models (Freud, 1900, 1923) conceived of the mind as an arena for competing internal forces – drives, phantasies, and defences. In this view, the internal world was primarily shaped by the individual's struggle to manage biological impulses (the id) against the constraints of reality and morality (the ego and superego).

While these models provided a revolutionary map of human interiority, they were essentially "one-person" psychologies. The environment – the actual, lived relationship between the child and the caregiver – was often viewed merely as the stage upon which these internal drives played out. Trauma, in this early framework, was often reduced to the frustration of a drive or the failure of a defence. For the modern clinician working with the long-term effects of relational neglect, this model can feel strangely empty of the other.

By the 1940s, this intrapsychic focus came into a productive, if fierce, collision. The "Controversial Discussions" within the British Psychoanalytical Society (1942–1944) were more than just institutional politics;

they represented a fundamental disagreement over the origins of the internal world. On one side stood Anna Freud (1946), who maintained the importance of drive theory and the adaptive functions of the ego, viewing the internal world as a structure built to manage the pressures of reality. On the other stood Melanie Klein (1932, 1948), who began to populate the internal world with "internal objects" – primitive, often terrifying mental representations derived from the infant's earliest experiences.

Klein's work moved the needle towards the relational by suggesting that the infant is in a constant, phantasy-driven relationship with objects (such as the mother's breast). However, for the clinician interested in the impact of *actual* caregiving, the limitation of the Kleinian model is its tendency to privilege the infant's innate, constitutional aggression (the death instinct) over environmental reality. In the Kleinian internal world, the "bad object" is often a projection of the infant's own rage, rather than a reflection of a truly failing parent. To bridge the gap towards a theory of cumulative relational trauma we required a perspective that took the environment seriously.

The Relational Turn: The Independent Tradition and the Primacy of the Other

The real shift towards the themes of this volume – attachment, environment, and the subtle disruptions of the self – was spearheaded by the Middle Group or Independents. Thinkers such as Ronald Fairbairn, Donald Winnicott, and Michael Balint challenged the very core of Freudian drive theory, suggesting that the human condition is fundamentally social.

Fairbairn (1952) made the revolutionary claim that the libido is not "pleasure-seeking" but "object-seeking". We do not reach out to others merely to satisfy a biological itch or to discharge tension; we reach out because we are inherently programmed to connect. In this framework, the internal world is formed when the child is forced to internalise unsatisfactory or rejecting objects as a way of managing environmental failure. By taking the badness of the parent into themselves, the child preserves the hope that the parent is actually good, and that they themselves are the source of the trouble. This "moral defence" is a cornerstone of our understanding of cumulative trauma: the internal world becomes a compensatory structure, a way of surviving what was missing or damaging in the external world.

Donald Winnicott (1958, 1965) took this further with his famous declaration that "there is no such thing as an infant" – only an infant and a mother. His work shifted the clinical focus entirely to the *quality of care* provided by the "holding environment". When a mother is "good-enough", she provides a space where the infant can simply be. But when the environment fails to provide this holding – through chronic misattunement or psychological intrusion – the child is forced to develop a "false self". This false self is a defensive facade, a relational mask designed to protect the "true self" from further fragmentation.

In these Independent thinkers we see the first clear outlines of the procedural past. They recognised that the internal world is not just a collection of conscious memories but a set of defensive manoeuvres and relational patterns. The internal world is where the child's attempt to survive their environment is stored. This transition from drive to relation allows us to see the patient not as a victim of their own impulses but as a survivor of their relational history. The formation of this procedural past, and its roots in early caregiver–infant interaction, is explored empirically and clinically through infant observation in Chapter 3.

If the Independents shifted psychoanalysis toward the primacy of the relational environment, developmental researchers provided the empirical detail that showed how this environment is internalised moment by moment.

Developmental Foundations: The Vulnerability of the Emerging Self

While the shift from drive to relation provided the theoretical scaffolding for a new psychoanalysis, it was the work of developmental researchers that provided the granular detail of how the internal world is constructed in real-time. Thinkers such as Margaret Mahler (Mahler et al., 1975) and the Tysons (Tyson & Tyson, 1990) offered maps of the child's journey from the undifferentiated state of infancy towards a cohesive sense of self. However, for the clinician working with relational trauma these developmental milestones are not merely academic stages; they represent critical windows of vulnerability where the internal world can become fractured.

Mahler's concept of the "separation-individuation" process describes the child's psychological birth. It is a journey that moves from the normal symbiosis of early infancy – where the child experiences no boundary between self and other – through the sub-phases of hatching, practising, and rapprochement. In a healthy environment, the caregiver acts as a secure base, allowing the child to venture out into the world and return for "emotional refuelling". This rhythmic movement between autonomy and connection is the process by which a resilient internal world is built.

Yet, when we examine these stages through the lens of cumulative trauma, we see how easily this process can be derailed. If a caregiver is unable to tolerate the child's growing autonomy, or conversely, if they withdraw emotionally when the child seeks proximity, the rapprochement phase becomes a site of chronic anxiety. The child's internal world begins to encode a fundamental conflict: that to be independent is to be abandoned, or to be close is to be engulfed. By re-centring Mahler's work within a relational framework, we move away from a pedagogical checklist of behaviours and towards a deeper understanding of how the internal world is shaped by the caregiver's own capacity for affect regulation.

The Tysons (Tyson & Tyson, 1990) furthered this integration by suggesting that development is not a linear progression but a complex, multidimensional system. They highlighted how different "lines of development" – affective, cognitive, and social – interweave. For the clinician, this means that a patient may be highly sophisticated in their cognitive understanding of their history, yet remain procedurally stuck at a much earlier affective level. This developmental asynchrony is a hallmark of cumulative trauma, where the internal world is a patchwork of advanced defences and primitive, unregulated fears.

These developmental insights set the stage for the next major evolution: the recognition that early relational patterns are not simply remembered but encoded as procedural templates that guide future relationships.

The Procedural Past: Attachment and the Archive of the Body

The most robust empirical bridge between the internal world and the external environment was built by John Bowlby. Disenchanted by the intrapsychic focus of his contemporaries, Bowlby (1997, 1998a, 1998b) turned to ethology and systems theory to explain the biological necessity of the attachment bond. He proposed that the infant is biologically programmed to seek proximity to a caregiver under conditions of threat. This is not a search for pleasure, as Freud suggested, but a search for safety.

Out of these early interactions, the child constructs what Bowlby termed internal working models (IWMs). These are mental representations of the self, the other, and the relationship between the two. These models are the blueprints of the internal world; they provide the templates through which all future relational data is filtered. A secure IWM tells the child: "I am worthy of care, and others are dependable." An insecure IWM, forged in the heat of cumulative trauma, tells the child: "I must hide my needs to stay safe, or I must be loud and demanding to be seen."

The revolutionary shift in our understanding of these models came with the recognition that they are stored in procedural memory. While declarative or narrative memory allows us to recall facts and events of our lives, procedural memory holds the "how" of our relational lives. As researchers such as Mary Main (Main et al., 1985) and the Boston Change Process Study Group (2002) have demonstrated, these procedural patterns are encoded long before the hippocampus – responsible for narrative memory – is fully functional.

This means that the internal world is, in large part, an archive of the body. It is what Christopher Bollas (1987) so evocatively called the "unthought known". These are relational truths that have been experienced and encoded but have never reached the level of symbolic thought. In the clinical setting, these procedural memories are not recalled through speech; they are *enacted* in the transference-countertransference matrix. How these bodily and affective archives reappear within the therapeutic relationship, and how they may be transformed through relational process, is taken up in Chapter 9.

For the patient who has suffered cumulative trauma, the internal world is often populated by these unthought procedural ghosts. They may feel a pervasive sense of shame or a chronic expectation of rejection without being able to link these feelings to a specific event. The trauma is not a memory in the traditional sense; it is a way of being. Therefore, the therapeutic work must go beyond the interpretation of content. It must involve the re-organisation of these procedural patterns through the lived experience of the therapeutic relationship – a process of moving from enactment to mentalisation, or the capacity to think about feelings (Fonagy et al., 2002).

Attachment theory opened the door to understanding the procedural past; contemporary neuroscience walked through it, revealing the biological mechanisms through which these early patterns are inscribed in the brain.

The Social Brain: Neurobiological Integration and the Architecture of Affect

To bridge the gap between early psychoanalytic intuition and twenty-first-century clinical reality, we must look at how the internal world is physically mapped within the human nervous system. Contemporary neuroscience – most notably the work of Allan Schore (2003, 2012) and Louis Cozolino (2002) – has provided a biological substrate for what the Independent tradition and attachment theorists suggested decades ago: that the mind is a relational organ.

The human brain is not a finished product at birth; it is a social organ that is sculpted by the relational environment. The right hemisphere, which is dominant for the first two to three years of life, is specifically designed to process non-verbal communication, emotional expression, and the sense of self. It is within these right-brain structures – the limbic system and the orbitofrontal cortex – that the internal world resides. In a healthy, secure attachment, right-brain-to-right-brain communication between the caregiver and the infant allows for the mutual regulation of high-arousal states. The caregiver acts as an external regulator for the infant's developing nervous system, essentially lending their mature brain to the child to help manage stress.

However, when we consider cumulative trauma, this neurobiological perspective becomes crucial. Cumulative relational trauma is not necessarily defined by a single catastrophic event, but by a chronic lack of affective resonance or regulation. If a caregiver is consistently unavailable, frightened, or intrusive, the infant's right brain is flooded with stress hormones like cortisol, which can have a lasting impact on the architecture of the brain. The internal world of the traumatised patient is thus often a physiologically disorganised one. These patients do not just think they are unsafe; their nervous systems are perpetually caught in a state of hyper-arousal or dissociative shutdown.

This neurobiological integration transforms our understanding of the clinical encounter. It suggests that the "talking cure" must fundamentally be a "feeling cure". Because the trauma is encoded in subcortical, right-brain structures that operate beneath the level of language, intellectual insight alone is often insufficient for change. The therapeutic relationship must serve as a neurobiological laboratory where the clinician provides the regulation that was missing in childhood. Through the medium of the transference and the clinician's own right-brain receptivity (countertransference), we work to foster new neural pathways, moving the patient from a state of physiological reactivity to one of emotional reflection.

Once we understand how relational experience shapes the architecture of the brain, the intergenerational dimension becomes unavoidable: the caregiver's own history is carried forward not only through narrative but through affective and neurobiological pathways.

The Intergenerational Web: Ghosts and Ancestors

The exploration of the social brain inevitably leads us beyond the individual to the historical family system. If the internal world is a relational construct, it is also an intergenerational one. As Selma Fraiberg famously described, there are "ghosts in the nursery" (Fraiberg et al., 1975) – unprocessed traumas and unresolved losses from the parents' own pasts that haunt the current relationship with the infant. Holmes (1999) has extended the metaphor from an attachment perspective to describe *ancestral ghosts* – unresolved attachment experiences and relational legacies that are transmitted across generations. These implicit patterns shape adult relational expectations and therapeutic enactments.

In the context of cumulative trauma, these ghosts are transmitted affectively rather than narratively. Through the work on disorganised attachment (Main & Hesse, 1990; Lyons-Ruth, 1999), we can observe how a parent's unresolved trauma creates a frightened or frightening presence. When the infant seeks safety in the caregiver but finds instead a source of alarm, they are placed in a biological paradox: the person they must flee from is the very person they must flee to. This "fright without solution" leads to a fragmented internal world where the self is experienced as fundamentally broken or bad.

This volume argues that much of what we encounter in the consulting room is the result of this intergenerational transmission. The unthought known of the parent – the trauma they could not name or process – becomes the procedural template for the child. However, alongside the malign ghosts, there are also benign ancestors – the resilient relational patterns, the good-enough moments, and the inherited strengths that provide the potential for healing.

By recognising the intergenerational nature of the internal world, the clinician can help the patient engage in a process of psychic sorting. We work to identify which aspects of the patient's internal experience are truly their own, and which are the projections of previous generations. This work is not merely about excavating the past; it is about reclaiming the present.

By bringing these intergenerational ghosts into the light of the therapeutic relationship, we allow them to be mourned and eventually laid to rest, freeing the patient to develop a more authentic and integrated sense of self.

Taken together, these strands of theory – from the intrapsychic to the intersubjective, from the developmental to the neurobiological, from the personal to the intergenerational – point towards a way of working that is neither reductionistic nor eclectic, but integrative in the deepest sense.

What unifies the chapters in this volume is an integrative stance that refuses the false choice between the intrapsychic and the relational. The internal world is understood here as both biologically grounded and intersubjectively shaped, a dynamic system in which early procedural patterns meet the possibilities of the present relationship. This perspective is neither a new school nor a hybrid of existing ones; it is a clinical posture that privileges curiosity, mutuality, and the transformative potential of affective experience. It is this stance – theoretically robust yet clinically humble – that forms the backbone of the work that follows.

Conclusion

This introductory chapter has sought to reframe the internal world as a dynamic, neurobiologically grounded, and relationally shaped space. We have traced the trajectory from the intrapsychic focus of classical theory to the environmental and relational focus of the Independent tradition, and finally to the empirical validation provided by attachment research and contemporary neuroscience.

The chapters that follow are organised to move the reader progressively from theory to clinical application. Part I examines the foundations of the internal world through attachment, developmental theory, and the procedural past. Part II turns to the clinical encounter, exploring how cumulative trauma is enacted and transformed within the therapeutic relationship. Part III widens the lens to consider intergenerational transmission and the broader relational field. Together, these sections offer an integrative framework for understanding how the internal world is formed, maintained, and ultimately reshaped in treatment. Part IV brings these strands together, offering integrative reflections on clinical practice and the wider implications for contemporary psychoanalytic work. This structure mirrors the clinical journey itself: from origins, to encounter, to transformation, and finally to integration.

The aim is to invite the reader into a way of working that is both theoretically robust and clinically humble. The chapters are not meant to be definitive answers, but rather retrospective reflections of a clinical journey – a journey that recognises that the internal world is a vast territory where healing is always possible through the power of the relational encounter. If such an integrative perspective is to be clinically useful, it must be grounded in an understanding of how relational experience is first organised developmentally.

References

Balint, M. (1968). *The basic fault: Therapeutic aspects of regression*. London: Tavistock Publications.

Bollas, C. (1987). *The shadow of the object: Psychoanalysis of the unthought known*. London: Free Association Books.

Boston Change Process Study Group. (2002). Forms of relational meaning: Issues in the relations between the implicit and reflective–verbal domains. *Infant Mental Health Journal*, 23(3), 247–269.

Bowlby, J. (1997). *Attachment and loss, vol. 1. Attachment*. London: Pimlico.

Bowlby, J. (1998a). *Attachment and loss, vol. 2. Separation: Anxiety and anger*. London: Pimlico.

Bowlby, J. (1998b). *Attachment and loss, vol. 3. Loss: sadness and depression*. London: Pimlico.

Cozolino, L. J. (2002). *The Neuroscience of psychotherapy: Building and rebuilding the human brain*. New York: W. W. Norton & Company.

Fairbairn, W. R. D. (1952). *Psychoanalytic studies of the personality*. London: Tavistock Publications.

Fonagy, P., Gergely, G., Jurist, E. L. & Target, M. (2002). *Affect regulation, mentalization, and the development of the self*. New York: Other Press.

Fraiberg, S., Adelson, E. & Shapiro, V. (1975). Ghosts in the nursery: A psychoanalytic approach to the problems of impaired infant–mother relationships. *Journal of the American Academy of Child Psychiatry*, 14(3), 387–421.

Freud, A. (1946). *The psychoanalytical treatment of children*. London: Imago Publishing Co.

Freud, S. (1900). The interpretation of dreams. In J. Strachey (ed.), *The standard edition of the complete psychological works of Sigmund Freud*, vols. 4–5. London: Hogarth Press.

Freud, S. (1923). The ego and the id. In J. Strachey (ed.), *The standard edition of the complete psychological works of Sigmund Freud*, vol. 19. London: Hogarth Press.

Holmes, J. (1999). Ghosts in the consulting room: An attachment perspective on intergenerational transmission. *Attachment & Human Development*, 1(1), 115–131.

Klein, M. (1932). *The psycho-analysis of children*. London: Hogarth Press.

Klein, M. (1948). *Contributions to psycho-analysis, 1921–1945*. London: Hogarth Press.

Lyons-Ruth, K. (1999). The two-person unconscious: Intersubjective dialogue, enactive representation, and the emergence of new forms of relational organization. *Psychoanalytic Inquiry*, 19(4), 576–617.

Mahler, M. S., Pine, F. & Bergman, A. (1975). *The Psychological Birth of the Human Infant*. New York: Basic Books.

Main, M. & Hesse, E. (1990). Parents' unresolved traumatic experiences are related to infant disorganized attachment status. In M. Greenberg, D. Cicchetti & E. Cummings (Eds.), *Attachment in the preschool years* (pp. 161–182). Chicago: University of Chicago Press.

Main, M., Kaplan, N. & Cassidy, J. (1985). Security in infancy, childhood, and adulthood: A move to the level of representation. *Monographs of the Society for Research in Child Development*, 50(1–2),66–104.

Schore, A. N. (2003). *Affect dysregulation and disorders of the self*. New York: W. W. Norton & Company.

Schore, A. N. (2012). *The science of the art of psychotherapy*. New York: W. W. Norton & Company.

Tyson, P. & Tyson, R. L. (1990). *Psychoanalytic theories of development: An integration*. New Haven, CT: Yale University Press.

Winnicott, D. W. (1958). *Collected papers: Through paediatrics to psycho-analysis*. London: Tavistock Publications.

Winnicott, D. W. (1965). *The maturational processes and the facilitating environment*. London: Hogarth Press.

2 Attachment, Security, Separation, and Psychological Differentiation

Developmental Implications

Retrospective Reflection

Looking back across the terrain of this chapter, what becomes most striking is the profound continuity between the infant's earliest relational experiences and the adult's later struggles with intimacy, autonomy, and affective coherence. The patterns that first emerge in the preverbal, right--brain-mediated domain do not simply fade with time; they become the implicit templates through which the individual anticipates, interprets, and organises relational life. The false self, the basic fault, the fear of breakdown, and the difficulties of separation–individuation all represent attempts to manage developmental environments that could not sustain the child's spontaneous gesture or tolerate their emerging difference.

Yet the chapter also points towards the possibility of transformation. Just as early relationships shape the developing mind, later relationships – particularly therapeutic ones – can reopen pathways that were foreclosed, symbolise experiences that were never represented, and restore capacities that were once split off or muted. The developmental story is not fixed; it is revisited in every meaningful encounter. In this sense, the therapeutic relationship becomes a second chance at psychological birth, offering the individual the opportunity to experience safety, recognition, and differentiation in ways that were previously unavailable.

Introduction

Early relational experience forms the matrix within which the infant's sense of security, emotional coherence, and emerging selfhood take shape. The caregiver's capacity to recognise, regulate, and respond to the infant's affective states provides the foundation for what Bowlby (1997) described as "felt security": a state of mind that enables the child to explore, to tolerate frustration, and to begin differentiating self from other. When this matrix is stable and attuned, it supports the gradual emergence of autonomy, psychological differentiation, and the capacity to engage the world as an agentic subject. When it is inconsistent, intrusive, or inverted – when the

DOI: 10.4324/9781003789727-4

child is recruited into meeting the caregiver's emotional needs – the developmental trajectory is altered in ways that reverberate across the lifespan.

This chapter traces the developmental arc through which attachment, separation, and differentiation unfold, integrating perspectives from attachment theory, object relations, separation–individuation theory, and contemporary neurobiology. We begin by examining the early attachment relationship as the primary organiser of the infant's emotional life, before turning to the defensive structures that arise when this relationship is distorted, including the false self and the basic fault. We then explore the child's movement towards autonomy through the lens of separation–individuation, highlighting the caregiver's role in supporting the child's "aggressive gesture" and tolerating difference. These psychological processes are then situated within the neurobiological findings that show how early relational patterns become encoded in implicit memory and right-brain circuitry, shaping affect regulation and vulnerability to cumulative trauma. The memory systems through which these early relational patterns are encoded and carried forward – often outside conscious awareness – are explored in greater depth in Chapter 6.

The chapter also considers the role of the father – or more broadly, the third position – in supporting differentiation, triangulation, and the development of mentalisation. The presence or absence of this third relational anchor has profound implications for the child's capacity to negotiate separation without fear of annihilation, and to develop a coherent, reflective sense of self. Finally, we draw together these threads to consider the developmental pathways that lead from early relational disturbance to later psychopathology, and the protective potential of secure attachment relationships across the lifespan.

By following this developmental trajectory, the chapter establishes the foundations for understanding how early relational experience shapes the architecture of the mind, and how therapeutic work later in life reactivates and reorganises these formative patterns. It sets the stage for the subsequent chapters, which examine trauma, mentalisation, and the processes through which psychological change becomes possible.

The developmental story begins with the infant's earliest relational environment. Before questions of autonomy, differentiation, or defiance can emerge, the child must experience a reliable sense of emotional safety. Attachment theory provides the conceptual foundation for understanding how this sense of security is transmitted, and how early relational patterns organise the infant's capacity to regulate affect and engage the world.

Foundation of Felt Security

Data from developmental studies show that in the earliest period of life the primary mechanism for transmitting a sense of security and coherence – or, conversely, insecurity and disorganisation – is the quality of the infant–

caregiver relationship. The caregiver's capacity to recognise, regulate, and respond to the infant's affective states establishes the foundation for what Bowlby (1997, 1998) conceptualised as felt security. When this matrix is stable and attuned, the infant internalises a sense of emotional continuity that supports exploration, curiosity, and the gradual emergence of self-organisation.

Bowlby (1979) emphasised that this relational matrix is easily disrupted when the caregiver seeks emotional security from the child, thereby inverting the caregiving hierarchy. A parent who recruits the child into providing comfort or stability – often in the context of relational conflict or inadequate support – places the child in a developmentally untenable position. Such relational inversion is associated with later attachment disturbances and difficulties in affect regulation. As Bowlby (1979) observed, children who are drawn into caring for a parent or younger siblings may grow into adults who carry a latent yearning for care, alongside dysregulated anger towards the parents who failed to provide it, and guilt or shame for expressing such needs.

Sroufe and Waters (1977) further highlight that the child's sense of felt security vitally affects their capacity to tolerate separation and to explore the environment without becoming overwhelmed by fear. The caregiver's provision of a secure base and safe haven enables the child to move between proximity and exploration, establishing the early template for negotiating connection and autonomy. Implicit in attachment theory, therefore, is the idea that separation is only unproblematic when attachment is secure.

When the attachment matrix is sufficiently attuned, the child internalises a sense of emotional continuity that supports exploration and emerging autonomy. But when the caregiver is unable to provide this stability – whether through emotional unavailability, inconsistency, or the inversion of the caregiving hierarchy – the child must adapt in ways that protect the relationship at the cost of the self. The theories of Winnicott, Balint, and Bowlby illuminate how such adaptations crystallise into defensive organisations that shape later patterns of relating and self-experience. These chronic relational adaptations form the developmental groundwork for what will later be conceptualised as cumulative relational trauma, a framework developed in detail in Chapter 5.

Distortions of Early Relational Experience – False Self and Basic Fault

Commenting on Winnicott's (1960) theory of emotional development, Bowlby (1979) suggests that relational environments in which the child is required to meet the caregiver's emotional needs generate what Winnicott termed a "false self" organisation. In such contexts, the child suppresses spontaneous gestures and authentic emotional expression in order to maintain the caregiver's stability. The discovery of the "true self", Bowlby argues, involves helping the person recognise and own their yearning for love and care, and to express the anger felt toward those who earlier failed to provide it – in essence, to mourn the loss of what was needed but not received.

Balint (1979) offers a parallel formulation. He proposes that a serious discrepancy between the infant's early needs and the care available creates a "deficiency state", later experienced phenomenologically as a "basic fault". Individuals who carry this early deficit often develop tenuous object relations and may attempt to compensate for the absence of inner wellbeing through self-destructive behaviours involving alcohol, drugs, or food. These behaviours can be understood as attempts to regulate affect in the absence of an internalised sense of safety.

Across these perspectives, a common theme emerges: when the caregiver cannot provide a reliable emotional environment, the child adapts by constricting authentic expression and organising the self around compliance, vigilance, or premature caregiving. These adaptations preserve the relationship but compromise the child's capacity for spontaneity, agency, and emotional integration. They also set the stage for later difficulties in negotiating separation and individuation, as the child has learned that autonomy threatens the stability of the relational field.

The Process of Separation–Individuation

Mahler et al.'s (1985) separation–individuation framework offers a complementary vantage point on the developmental challenges that arise when early caregiving is distorted. From this perspective, the infant's movement toward autonomy depends on the caregiver's capacity to tolerate the child's emerging difference – emotionally, physically, and psychologically. When the caregiver cannot bear this differentiation, the child's developmental trajectory becomes constrained in ways that echo throughout later life.

Mahler and Furer (1967) observed that when a caregiver relates to the infant in a manner that is too exclusive and too parasitic, the child may experience separation as catastrophic rather than developmental. In such contexts, the infant's attempts to move away – literally or symbolically – evoke intense anxiety, sometimes resembling the annihilation dread seen in adult psychosis. Later work by Mahler and colleagues (Mahler et al., 1985) elaborated that psychological differentiation is impeded both when the caregiver keeps the child in a dependent position to meet their own emotional needs, and when the caregiver prematurely pushes the child towards autonomy without adequate emotional support. In both scenarios, the child's emerging sense of self is compromised.

For separation–individuation to unfold optimally, the caregiver must remain emotionally available while allowing the child to explore, assert, and experiment with autonomy. This relational stance enables the infant to experience themselves and the caregiver as distinct subjects – each with their own intentions, affects, and perspectives. When this process is supported, the child internalises a sense of agency and coherence that becomes foundational for later psychological resilience.

Khan (1979), drawing on Winnicott's (1960, 1974) object-relational formulations, emphasises that the caregiver's own conflicts can severely disrupt this developmental process. When the caregiver cannot tolerate the child's "aggressive gesture" – the spontaneous assertion of will, desire, or frustration – the child is forced to split off these vital aspects of self. Rage, defiance, and protest become dangerous because they threaten the caregiver's stability. The child learns to mute or disavow these impulses, resulting in a depleted sense of self and a constriction of spontaneity. Winnicott's (1960) observation that the child "ceases to exist" when their spontaneous gesture is not met finds poignant expression here.

Khan further argues that a merged or enmeshed maternal style undermines the development of what Winnicott (1958) termed "the capacity to be alone" – the ability to feel secure in one's own company without fear of abandonment or collapse. This difficulty is compounded when a father or third relational figure is absent or emotionally unavailable. In such relational configurations, the mother's eventual withdrawal from the intense dyadic bond is experienced not as a natural step in development but as a traumatic rupture. The child is left with a pervasive sense of impending catastrophe – a state Winnicott (1974) famously described as the "fear of a breakdown that has already happened" but has not yet been consciously experienced or symbolised.

Across these perspectives, a coherent picture emerges: the child's capacity for separation, autonomy, and psychological differentiation depends on a relational environment that can tolerate aggression, defiance, and difference. When this environment is compromised – through enmeshment, inconsistency, or the caregiver's own unmet needs – the child's developmental momentum is diverted. The result is a fragile sense of self, difficulties with affect regulation, and a chronic fear of abandonment or collapse that may persist into adulthood.

A Neurobiological Perspective

Contemporary neurobiological research deepens our understanding of why early relational disturbances exert such enduring effects. Traumatic or dysregulated caregiving environments shape the developing brain through implicit, non-verbal channels that precede the maturation of declarative memory. When the infant is repeatedly exposed to fear, inconsistency, or emotional unavailability, these experiences become encoded in right--hemisphere circuits responsible for affect regulation, stress responsivity, and the organisation of implicit relational expectations.

Findings from trauma and memory research suggest that the difficulty many individuals have in consciously recalling early traumatic states reflects the nature of implicit encoding rather than an absence of impact. The infant's nervous system registers cumulative threat long before it can symbolise or narrate experience. As a result, later states of fear, collapse, or dysregulation may be rooted in early relational trauma that has never been consciously represented. This implicit imprinting is consistent with clinical presentations associated with disorganised attachment, in which the caregiver is simultaneously a source of comfort *and* fear (Main & Hesse, 1990). Neurobiological studies (Perry et al., 1995; van der Kolk, 1994; Schacter, 1996) similarly show that repeated activation of stress circuits can lead to enduring alterations in arousal, attention, and affective integration.

From this perspective, the "fear of a breakdown" described by Winnicott (1974) can be understood as the somatic echo of early relational trauma that has not been symbolised. The individual may live with a pervasive sense of impending catastrophe, not because a breakdown is imminent, but because the nervous system continues to register an unintegrated past. Therapeutic work often involves helping the individual bring these implicit states into relational and bodily awareness, allowing them to be experienced, named, and gradually reorganised within a secure interpersonal context.

Cumulative Trauma

Khan's (1979) concept of cumulative trauma provides a powerful lens for understanding how chronic relational disturbances shape the developing self. Rather than focusing on discrete traumatic events, Khan emphasises the pathogenic impact of persistent relational patterns – particularly those in which the caregiver cannot support the child's movement towards separation and psychological differentiation. When the caregiver's needs dominate the relational field, the child's emerging autonomy is experienced as dangerous or forbidden. Over time, this dynamic fosters self-alienation, identity diffusion, and a chronic sense of internal disorganisation. These dynamics do not remain confined to childhood.

Stoller (1986) and Stubrin (1994) similarly argue that when the child's sense of self is endangered by relational intrusions or failures, defensive strategies may become sexualised in adulthood. These authors highlight that sexualised enactments can function as attempts to manage dissociated hatred, fear, or longing – affects that could not be expressed or metabolised within the early caregiving relationship. Litowitz (2002) extends this view by suggesting that non-sexual defensive motivations may take on sexualised forms when the individual's core sense of self is under threat. This echoes Freud's (1918) concept of *Nachträglichkeit* – a rearrangement or re-transcription of past experience in a context of new circumstances.

Across these perspectives, aggression and defiance emerge as essential developmental capacities. They signal the child's movement towards separateness and the assertion of a subjective perspective. When these impulses are suppressed – because they threaten the caregiver or destabilise the relational field – the child's capacity for autonomous exploration is compromised. As Benjamin (1992) and Ogden (1986) note, without the recognition of difference, subjectivity cannot fully emerge. These dynamics often reappear in adolescence, when the "second individuation process" (Blos, 1962) reactivates earlier struggles around autonomy, defiance, and relational negotiation.

The Role of the Father

A growing body of psychoanalytic and developmental literature underscores the importance of the father – or more broadly, a third relational figure – in supporting the child's movement towards differentiation. Campbell (1999) and Fonagy and Target (1999) argue that the father's presence introduces a third perspective that disrupts the intensity of the mother–child dyad, offering the child a relational alternative and a pathway towards triangulation. This third position provides a psychological space in which the child can experience themselves as separate from both parents, facilitating the development of mentalisation.

Panksepp's (2001) neurobiological research adds a further dimension. He suggests that rough-and-tumble play – often characteristic of father–child interactions – supports the maturation of frontal lobe circuits involved in emotional regulation, impulse control, and social communication. Deprivation of such playful engagement may contribute to developmental delays associated with emotional and behavioural difficulties, including ADHD. This view aligns with the work of Schore (1994, 2001), Siegel (2001), and Trevarthen (2001), who emphasise that early relational experiences shape the neural architecture underlying self-regulation, intersubjectivity, and the capacity to share emotional meaning.

Despite the developmental significance of fathers, many children grow up with fathers who are physically absent or emotionally unavailable. Contemporary social conditions – long working hours, high rates of separation and divorce – exacerbate this absence. When the child's attachment to both parents is compromised, the risk of serious psychopathology increases unless a protective attachment is available elsewhere in the family system. As Holmes (2001) notes, even a single secure relationship – such as with a grandparent or aunt – can buffer the effects of early relational trauma. Fonagy et al. (1997) similarly argue that secure attachment provides the intersubjective foundation for mentalisation, enabling the child to reflect on and eventually resolve traumatic experience. Such protective relationships may divert the developmental trajectory away from borderline personality disorder and other severe psychopathologies (Bradley, 2003).

Conclusion

Taken together, these developmental perspectives illuminate how the infant's earliest relational environment shapes the architecture of the mind. Secure attachment provides the emotional scaffolding from which autonomy, affect regulation, and psychological differentiation can emerge. When this matrix is disrupted – through inconsistency, enmeshment, relational inversion, or the caregiver's own unresolved conflicts – the child adapts in ways that preserves the relationship but compromises the self. These adaptations become woven into implicit memory, right-brain circuitry, and the defensive organisations that structure later patterns of relating. How these early relational patterns are reactivated and worked with in the therapeutic relationship is examined in Chapter 9.

This chapter has traced how these early relational dynamics reverberate across the lifespan, influencing vulnerability to cumulative trauma, shaping the capacity for mentalisation, and determining whether separation is experienced as growth or annihilation. The presence of a third relational figure, particularly the father, can provide a vital counterbalance, offering the child a triangulated space in which difference, agency, and mentalisation can develop. These developmental pathways form the foundation for understanding how therapeutic work later in life reactivates, revisits, and reorganises these early patterns, opening the possibility for new forms of emotional experience and relational engagement. Infant observation offers one of the few ways of apprehending these processes as they unfold, before they become organised into narrative or defensive structure.

References

Balint, M. (1979). *The basic fault*. London: Routledge.

Benjamin, J. (1992). Recognition and destruction: An outline of intersubjectivity. In J. Benjamin, *Like subjects, love objects: Essays on recognition and sexual difference* (pp. 27–48). New Haven, CT: Yale University Press.

Blos, P. (1962). The second individuation process of adolescence. In *On adolescence: A psychoanalytic interpretation* (pp. 77–101). London: Free Association Press.

Bowlby, J. (1997). *Attachment and loss, vol. 1. Attachment*. London: Pimlico.

Bowlby, J. (1998). *Attachment and loss, vol. 2. Separation: Anger and anxiety*. London: Pimlico.

Bowlby, J. (1979). *The making and breaking of affectional bonds*. London: Tavistock Publications.

Bradley, S. J. (2003). *Affect regulation and the development of psychopathology*. New York: Guilford Press.

Campbell, D. (1999). The role of the father in a pre-suicide state. In R. S. Perelberg (Ed.), *Psychoanalytic understanding of violence and suicide* (pp. 75–86). London: Routledge.

Fonagy, P., Steele, M., Steele, H., Higgitt, A. & Target, M. (1997). The theory and practice of resilience. *Journal of Child Psychology and Psychiatry*, 38(2), 231–257.

Fonagy, P. & Target, M. (1999). Towards understanding violence: The use of the body and the role of the father. In R. S. Perelberg (ed.), *Psychoanalytic understanding of violence and suicide* (pp. 53–72). London: Routledge.

Freud, S. (1918). From the history of an infantile neurosis. In J. Strachey (ed.), *The standard edition of the complete psychological works of Sigmund Freud*, vol. 17, 1–122. London: Hogarth Press.

Holmes, J. (2001). *The search for a secure base: Attachment theory and psychotherapy*. Hove: Brunner-Routledge.

Khan, M. (1979). *Alienation in perversions*. London: Karnac Books.

Litowitz, B. E. (2002). Sexuality and textuality. *Journal of the American Psychoanalytic Association*, 50(1), 171–198.

Mahler, M. S. & Furer, M. (1967). On human symbiosis and the vicissitudes of individuation: Infantile psychosis. *Journal of the American Psychoanalytic Association*, 15, 740–753.

Mahler, M. S., Pine, F. & Bergman, A. (1985). *The psychological birth of the human infant: Symbiosis and individuation*. London: Karnac Books.

Main, M. & Hesse, E. (1990). Parents' unresolved traumatic experiences are related to infant disorganized attachment status: Is frightened and/or frightening parental behaviour the linking mechanism? In M. Greenberg, D. Cicchetti & E. Cummings (Eds.), *Attachment in the preschool years: Theory, research and intervention* (pp. 161–182). Chicago, IL: University of Chicago Press.

Ogden, T. H. (1986). *The matrix of the mind: Object relations and the psychoanalytic dialogue*. Northvale, NJ: Jason Aronson.

Panksepp, J. (2001). The long-term psychobiological consequences of infant emotions: Prescriptions for the twenty-first century. *Infant Mental Health Journal*, 22, 132–173.

Perry, B. D., Pollard, R. A., Blakely, T. L., Baker, W. L. & Vigilante, D. (1995). Childhood trauma, the neurobiology of adaptation, and "use-dependent" development of the brain: How "states" become "traits". *Infant Mental Health Journal*, 16, 271–291.

Schacter, D. L. (1996). *Searching for memory: The brain, the mind, and the past*. New York: Basic Books.

Schore, A. N. (1994). *Affect regulation and the origin of the self: The neurobiology of emotional development*. Hillsdale, NJ: Lawrence Erlbaum Associates.

Schore, A. N. (2001). The effects of early relational trauma on right brain development, affect regulation and infant mental health. *Infant Mental Health Journal*, 22, 201–269.

Siegel, D. J. (2001). Toward an interpersonal neurology of the developing mind: Attachment relationships, "mindsight" and neural integration. *Infant Mental Health Journal*, 22, 67–94.

Sroufe, L. A. & Waters, E. (1977). Attachment as an organizational construct. *Child Development*, 48, 1184–1199.

Stern, D. N. (1985). *The interpersonal world of the infant: A view from psychoanalysis and developmental psychology*. New York: Basic Books.

Stern, D. N., Sander, L. W., Nahum, J. P., Harrison, A. M., Lyons-Ruth, K., Morgan, A. C., Bruschweiler-Stern, N. & Tronick, E. Z. (1998). The process of therapeutic change involving implicit knowledge: Some implications of developmental observations for adult psychotherapy. *Infant Mental Health Journal*, 19(3), 300–308.

Stoller, R. J. (1986). Perversion: The erotic form of hatred. *Journal of Child Psychology and Psychiatry*, 38 (2), 231–257.

Stubrin, J. P. (1994). *Sexualities and homosexualities*, (trans. E. Reneboldi). London: Karnac Books.

Trevarthen, C. (2001). Intrinsic motives for companionship in understanding: Their origin, development and significance for infant mental health. *Infant Mental Health Journal*, 22, 95–131.

van der Kolk, B. A. (1994). The body keeps the score: Memory and the evolving psychobiology of post-traumatic stress. *Harvard Review of Psychiatry*, 1, 253–265.

van der Kolk, B. A. & Fisler, R. (1995). Dissociation and the fragmentary nature of traumatic memories: Overview and exploratory study. *Journal of Traumatic Stress*, 8 (4), 505–521.

Winnicott, D. W. (1958). The capacity to be alone. *International Journal of Psycho-Analysis*, 39, 416–420.

Winnicott, D. W. (1960). Ego distortion in terms of true and false self. In *The maturational processes and the facilitating environment* (pp. 140–152). London: Hogarth Press.

Winnicott, D. W. (1974). Fear of breakdown. *International Review of Psycho-Analysis*, 1, 103–107.

3 The Procedural Past

Infant Observation and the Relational Foundations of Adult Psychotherapy

Retrospective Reflection

Looking back across the years, I can see how much of what now feels natural in my clinical work began in a far more tentative, embryonic form. When I first encountered infant observation, I did not yet have the language, the theoretical scaffolding, or even the confidence to understand what I was learning. What I did have was a sense – sometimes unsettling, sometimes quietly thrilling – that something important was happening in the space between observer and observed. I was being shaped by experiences I could not yet articulate.

In those early days, I often felt as though I was standing at the edge of a vast terrain, sensing its contours but unable to map them. I knew that the infant's world was organised through rhythms, gestures, and affective tides, but I did not yet grasp how deeply those same processes would later reveal themselves in the consulting room. I was learning to watch, to wait, to feel my way into another's experience without rushing to interpret. At the time, it felt like an apprenticeship in attentiveness. Only later did I realise it was also an apprenticeship in clinical presence.

As my practice developed, the implicit lessons of infant observation began to surface with greater clarity. I found myself listening not only to what patients said but to how they said it – the pauses, the hesitations, the shifts in tone that signalled something stirring beneath the surface. I recognised familiar patterns: the tentative reach for connection, the sudden withdrawal, the oscillation between hope and dread. These were not abstract concepts but living procedures, echoes of early relational life playing out in the therapeutic moment.

What had once been intuitive but unformulated gradually became explicit. I began to understand that the therapeutic encounter is shaped as much by implicit communication as by conscious thought. The patient's procedural past – their early ways of managing proximity, affect, and vulnerability – emerges in the room with a kind of quiet insistence. And my task, as I came to see it, was not simply to interpret these patterns but to meet them with a form of presence that could hold, regulate, and eventually transform them.

DOI: 10.4324/9781003789727-5

How the patient's procedural past emerges and is worked with through enactment in the therapeutic relationship is explored clinically in later chapters.

This shift in my clinical stance has been one of the most meaningful developments in my professional life. The observational discipline I learned years ago now feels woven into the fabric of my work. It guides the way I sit with patients, the way I listen, the way I allow myself to be affected. It reminds me that therapeutic change often begins before words are found – in the shared rhythms of attention, in the capacity to stay with what is unformulated, in the willingness to enter the patient's affective world without losing my own footing.

In this sense, infant observation has become more than a method; it has become a way of being with others. It has taught me that the past is not simply remembered but enacted, that the mind is shaped in relationship and reshaped in relationship, and that the clinician's presence can offer a new developmental possibility. The ideas that once felt elusive now feel lived. They have become part of the quiet, steady work of helping another person find new ways of relating – to themselves, to others, and to the world.

As the chapter unfolds, several moments from my infant observation experience illustrate how these early lessons in attunement, rupture, and repair became woven into my clinical sensibility. This may be seen in my work with Patricia (Chapter 9) and Katarina (Chapter 11).

Part I

Introduction: The Observational Stance and the Clinical Mind

Infant observation brings to life the deep continuity between early development and the developmental work of adult psychotherapy. This connection is especially salient given the high incidence of unresolved childhood trauma – neglect, loss, abuse – among those who seek treatment. What becomes visible through careful observation of the infant–caregiver dyad is the way micro-behavioural exchanges regulate affect and shape emerging patterns of relatedness. These same processes, transposed into the consulting room, form the substrate of therapeutic action.

Yet infant observation sits at a crossroads. It is taught as a phenomenological discipline in which the observer brackets theory and attends to lived experience with minimal interpretive interference. At the same time, contemporary developmental and relational research shows that even the simplest observational moment is already saturated with implicit meaning: micro-regulations of affect, mutual influence, procedural memory, and the early formation of relational schemas. The question is not whether theory informs observation – it inevitably does – but how to hold theory in suspension so that the observer can register experience before organising it into meaning. This chapter takes that tension as its point of departure, tracing the developmental and psychoanalytic traditions that have shaped observational practice and exploring their relevance for adult psychotherapy.

Relational Origins: Bowlby, Fairbairn, and the Primacy of Real Experience

Bowlby's (1998) reorientation of psychoanalysis towards real relationships remains foundational. He framed attachment as a biologically-based behavioural system through which the infant seeks proximity to a caregiver who provides safety and regulation. When this bond is disrupted through separation or loss, the infant experiences fear, dysregulation, and developmental derailment. Fairbairn's (1952) influence is unmistakable here: both theorists locate the origins of psychological structure in the infant's lived relational environment rather than in drive-based fantasy. Feelings of security or insecurity arise from actual interactions with caregivers and shape the organisation of internal object relations. Infant observation, in this light, becomes a method for witnessing the formation of these early relational templates.

Mahler and the Slow Emergence of Separateness

Mahler et al.'s (1985) account of early development centres on the infant's gradual movement from symbiotic attachment toward psychological differentiation. The phases of hatching, practising, and emotional refuelling unfold within a relational matrix in which the caregiver's attunement is crucial. Too much intrusion or too little availability can distort the infant's emerging sense of autonomy. Although Mahler's terminology differs from Bowlby's, both emphasise that confidence, exploration, and identity develop within a reliable relational environment. Infant observation makes these delicate negotiations visible in real time.

Affect, Trauma, and the Early Organisation of Mind: Tyson and Tyson

Tyson and Tyson (1990) integrate affect-trauma theory, ego psychology, self-psychology, and infant research to highlight the central role of affect in early psychological organisation. Through repeated interactions with an attuned caregiver, the infant links affective states with emerging ideas, memories, and fantasies. Affects gradually acquire a signal function, enabling the child to manage arousal rather than be overwhelmed by it. When parental empathy fails or trauma intrudes, this process is disrupted, compromising the development of a coherent sense of self. Their work underscores the developmental roots of the emotion-regulation difficulties so often encountered in adult psychotherapy.

Winnicott and the Holding of Experience

Winnicott's (1958, 1988) developmental vision centres on the mother's capacity to provide a holding environment in which the infant's experience can be organised and gradually integrated. Within this facilitating environment, the infant moves from subjective omnipotence towards an awareness of external reality, a transition supported by the mother's attuned responsiveness. Transitional phenomena – blankets, toys, rhythms of interaction – help the infant bridge the space between inner and outer worlds. A crucial aspect of the mother's role is her capacity to mirror the infant's experience, enabling the emergence of an authentic sense of self. When this process falters, the infant adapts prematurely to the mother's needs, compromising spontaneity and "true self" experience. The observational stance, in its receptive, non-intrusive quality, echoes Winnicott's vision of maternal presence.

Bion and the Transformation of Raw Experience

Bion's (1984) model of early development describes how raw sensory and emotional experiences – beta elements – are transformed into thinkable, meaningful content through the mother's capacity for reverie. In this state of receptive openness, the mother contains the infant's projections of fear, frustration, and unmanageable affect, metabolising them and returning them in a form the infant can tolerate. This container–contained process enables the infant to develop the capacity for thought, symbolisation, and emotional regulation. When the caregiver cannot perform this function, the infant is left with unprocessed emotional states that cannot be integrated. Bion's model highlights the deeply interactional nature of early mental life and underscores the importance of the observer's containing function during infant observation and later in adult psychotherapy.

Bollas and the Transformational Object

Bollas (1987) extends Winnicott and Bion by emphasising the mother as a transformational object – an early relational presence that shapes the infant's developing sense of being through countless micro-exchanges. These interactions convey the mother's implicit "theory of being", which the infant absorbs not through explicit teaching but through the lived experience of being with her. The infant brings an inherited disposition to these encounters, and together mother and child co-create the early architecture of subjective life. When the mother's implicit relational style is constraining or intrusive, the development of the infant's true self may be forestalled. Bollas's focus on the formative power of implicit relational processes resonates strongly with contemporary understandings of procedural memory, affective communication, and the micro-regulatory patterns that infant observation makes visible.

Attachment Research and the Shaping of Internal Worlds

Attachment research has consistently supported Bowlby's (1998) view that early relational experience shapes the infant's emerging internal world. Ainsworth's strange situation studies (Ainsworth et al., 1978; Ainsworth, 1982) demonstrated that patterns of secure, avoidant, ambivalent, and later disorganised attachment can be predicted from the quality of caregiver–infant interaction in the first year of life. These patterns become internal working models that guide attention, affect regulation, and expectations of others. Once established, they tend to be self-perpetuating, as information that contradicts the existing model may be defensively excluded or distorted.

Main and colleagues showed that a parent's sensitive responsiveness is the strongest predictor of secure attachment, whereas rejection, inconsistency, or frightened/frightening behaviour are associated with avoidant, ambivalent, and disorganised patterns (Main, 1991; Main & Hesse, 1990; Main et al., 1985). Disorganisation is particularly linked to maltreatment and unresolved trauma in the caregiver. Schore (1994) extends these findings by arguing that early psychopathology reflects failures of interactive and self-regulation of affect, rooted in disruptions to the attachment relationship.

Part II

The Infant as Active Partner: Empirical Studies of Early Interaction

Developmental research has shown that from the very beginning the infant is not a passive recipient of care but an active participant in relational life. Stern's (1985) synthesis of perceptual and behavioural studies demonstrates that the infant's systems are primed for social engagement; states of consciousness are shaped within ongoing interaction rather than arising in isolation. Tronick et al.'s (1978) still-face paradigm makes this vividly clear: when the caregiver suddenly becomes unresponsive, the infant's distress, protest, and eventual withdrawal reveal the centrality of attunement and the restorative power of repair.

Micro-analytic studies by Jaffe, Beebe, Lachmann and others (Beebe et al., 1985, 1992; Lachmann & Beebe, 1990; Jaffe et al., 2001) deepen this picture. They reveal the moment-to-moment coordination of gaze, vocal rhythm, movement, and affect between mother and infant. These patterns of timing, matching, and mutual influence form the basis of early affect regulation and are predictive of later attachment organisation and cognitive development. Over time, recurrent interaction patterns become internalised as procedural representations of "how relationships work", providing the foundation for later symbolic and relational capacities. Infant observation, with its disciplined attention to subtle shifts in rhythm and affect, offers a privileged vantage point from which to witness these processes as they unfold.

A natural way to deepen this discussion is to turn to a moment from my own infant-observation experience in which these micro-regulatory processes became vividly apparent. What struck me at the time was not simply the infant's responsiveness to the caregiver but the delicacy with which she modulated her own arousal through shifts in gaze, posture, and affective tone. In the space of a few seconds, one could see the dyad negotiating intensity, restoring equilibrium, and re-establishing connection. The following observation illustrates how these early forms of mutual regulation unfold in real time and how the infant's procedural repertoire is already shaping the relational field.

Observation 13

Imogen was in an alert state when I arrived, sucking her fingers. Bernie sat her sideways on her lap so she was face-to-face with me. Imogen smiled and met my gaze. I mirrored her facial expressions and added soft vocalisations. Although she made no sounds, she responded cross-modally by intensifying her gaze, widening her smile, and opening her mouth more fully. The affective intensity of our engagement gradually increased, culminating in a broad gape smile and prolonged visual regard.

After these moments of heightened mutual engagement, Imogen periodically looked away while remaining oriented face-to-face. She appeared to be using gaze aversion to regulate arousal. Each time she did so, I reduced the intensity of my stimulation, allowing her space to re-regulate. When she was ready, she re-engaged, and the cycle repeated several times. My own state mirrored hers: I felt a rising sense of pleasure and vitality. The matching of our behavioural displays, and the sense of mutual influence, seemed to generate a shared pleasurable state.

Later, while Bernie made coffee, I held Imogen face-to-face. Initially she showed a clear preference for Bernie, keeping her head turned to maintain their mutual gaze – an "invisible umbilical cord" of connection. After a while she turned back to me. I stood her up so she could flex her legs, occasionally lifting her. Her communication remained primarily kinesic: shifts in gaze, facial expression, and bodily movement. I found myself tracking and matching these movements through subtle changes in my vocal tone. Again, she regulated the intensity of the exchange by brief gaze aversions, and I adjusted accordingly. When she became more behaviourally active, I quietened; when she became still, I gently increased my stimulation. We seemed to share a rhythm, taking turns in a fluid, moment-to-moment "dialogue".

At one point, Imogen's gaze drifted leftward and took on a dreamy, inward quality. My vocalisations slowed and softened almost automatically, and I found myself saying, in a similarly dreamy tone, "There's a dreamy look." Observing her shift affected my own state, which became calm and reflective. I felt drawn to mirror her mood with a soft-focused gaze and gentle musicality. Bernie, watching, also seemed moved by the moment. It was another instance of Imogen regulating her own state while shaping the affective quality of our interaction.

Eventually our social play broke down. Imogen began to frown and became fretful, turning her head away from me towards Bernie. I handed her to Bernie, who immediately recognised that she was hungry and tired. She put Imogen to the breast and stroked her arm rhythmically. Imogen closed her eyes and soon fell into a deep sleep. Alongside tiredness, it seemed likely that she also needed to down-regulate after a long, intense period of social engagement. Imogen awoke shortly before I left, again alert and smiling, signalling readiness for more play. I felt a strong pull to stay and continue the interaction.

In relation to adult work, the observation highlights the importance of mirroring and matching between therapist and patient. Such behavioural symmetry provides a basis for sensing each other's rhythm and affective state. The therapist's own psychophysiological responses become an additional source of information about the patient's subjective experience. Turn-taking appears central to positive affective matching; when disrupted – for example, by talking over one another or misreading an intrapersonal pause as an interpersonal pause – the loss of contingency is felt as an impingement. If such patterns recur, they may indicate a re-enactment of entrenched internalised relational procedures.

As with the infant, gaze aversion in the adult may signal that the interaction has become too intense or anxiety-provoking. Sensitivity to such cues allows the patient space to self-regulate before re-engaging. This attuned, non-verbal responsiveness contributes to the creation of a holding environment and supports the development of a secure therapeutic alliance. Within such a setting, both transferential and developmental issues can be productively explored, organised, and integrated.

Misattunement, Withdrawal, and the Shaping of Self-regulation

Beebe, Jaffe and Lachmann (1992) describe misattunement as a breakdown in contingent responsiveness and mutual influence. When the infant repeatedly encounters non-contingent responses, negative affect and escalating arousal may follow, leading the infant to withdraw in order to self--regulate. Over time, such withdrawal can compromise attention, information processing, and the capacity to remain alert and engaged with the environment. Their work highlights how early dyadic patterns shape both interactive and self-regulatory capacities, and how these patterns may later be enacted in the therapeutic relationship.

An observation from this period of my training brought home the lived texture of such misattunements and their consequences. What had seemed, in theory, a straightforward description of non-contingency revealed itself in practice as a complex choreography of missed cues, rising frustration, and the infant's increasingly desperate attempts to restore a sense of connection. The mother's divided attention, though entirely understandable in context, created a momentary relational vacuum that the infant struggled to bridge. The vignette that follows captures the subtle but powerful impact of these micro-ruptures and the infant's efforts to regain a regulatory footing.

Observation 14

When I arrived, Imogen was lying on her back on the play mat. Bernie sat beside her, talking softly and stroking her tummy. Imogen responded with smiles and animated movements of her arms and legs. The interaction had a lively, mutually engaging rhythm. After a few minutes, however, Bernie's attention shifted towards her older daughter, who was preparing to leave for school. Although Bernie continued to speak intermittently to Imogen, her focus was divided.

Imogen's behaviour changed almost immediately. Her movements became more abrupt, her facial expression tightened, and she began to vocalise in short, sharp bursts. She seemed to be protesting the sudden drop in contingency. Bernie attempted to soothe her by offering a toy and speaking in a gentle tone, but her attention remained elsewhere. Imogen's distress escalated: she arched her back, kicked more vigorously, and her vocalisations took on a plaintive quality. The mismatch between her signals and Bernie's responses appeared to heighten her frustration.

When Bernie finally returned her full attention to Imogen, the infant's distress did not immediately subside. She turned her head away, avoiding Bernie's gaze, and her movements became disorganised. Bernie picked her up and held her close, rocking gently. Gradually, Imogen's body softened and her breathing slowed. After a short while she re-engaged, looking up at Bernie with a tentative smile. The dyad moved back into a more regulated rhythm, though the earlier rupture had left a residual fragility in the interaction.

A little later, during feeding, a similar pattern emerged. Imogen struggled at the breast, pulling away and fussing. Bernie tried to reposition her, but the interaction became a subtle battle of wills. Imogen's frustration mounted; she stiffened, turned her head, and vocalised in protest. Bernie persisted, attempting to guide her back to the breast. Eventually, after several minutes of dysregulated back-and-forth, Imogen settled and fed quietly. Once she had regained equilibrium, she gazed up at Bernie with a soft, open expression, and the tension dissipated.

Reflecting on the observation, what stood out was how quickly Imogen detected non-contingency and how powerfully it affected her regulatory capacity. The moment Bernie's attention shifted, the infant's arousal rose sharply, and her behaviour became increasingly disorganised. The subsequent repair required time, closeness, and sustained attunement. The feeding sequence echoed this dynamic: a brief mismatch escalated into a struggle, followed by a gradual return to synchrony.

In clinical terms, the observation illustrates how misattunement and rupture can activate early strategies for managing distress, and how the infant's attempts to restore connection may become entangled with emerging issues of control and frustration. The dyadic pattern – protest, escalation, withdrawal, and eventual repair – offers a vivid analogue to the relational sequences that often unfold in adult psychotherapy, particularly with patients whose early experiences were marked by inconsistency or noncontingency. The infant's rapid shifts between engagement and withdrawal highlight the fragility of early regulatory systems and the centrality of the caregiver's attuned presence in restoring balance. Such procedurally organised patterns often reappear as enactments within the therapeutic relationship, a process examined in detail in Chapter 10.

Stern and the Enduring Architecture of Relatedness

Stern's (1985) account of early development places the infant's subjective experience and interpersonal context at the centre. He proposes that the infant's emerging senses of self – emergent, core, subjective, and verbal – each open a corresponding domain of relatedness. These domains are not discrete phases but enduring modes of engagement that continue to organise relational life across the lifespan. Clinical issues such as autonomy, dependence, mastery, and separation are therefore not confined to infancy but recur throughout development in new forms.

Central to Stern's (1985) model is affect attunement: the caregiver's capacity to match the intensity, timing, and shape of the infant's affective states, often across sensory modalities. This attuned responsiveness provides the infant with a sense of coherence and continuity, enabling them to tolerate separations and regulate affect without resorting to defensive withdrawal. Stern (1985) sees these micro-regulatory exchanges as the building blocks of psychic structure, forming the perceptual, affective, and cognitive schemas through which later experience is organised.

These schemas take the form of procedural memories – nonconscious, non-verbalised patterns of "how we do things together". Repeated micro-events of mutual influence become generalised into what Stern (1985) terms "representations of interactions that have been generalised" (RIGs). RIGs precede and underpin the development of internal working models, providing the infant with a behavioural template for entering into the temporal and affective states of others.

One of my observations during this period offered a particularly clear window into the emergence of such expectancies. What unfolded between mother and infant was not simply a sequence of behaviours but a patterned exchange in which each partner anticipated the other's next move. The infant's gestures, vocalisations, and shifts in affect conveyed a nascent sense of agency, as though she were testing the reliability of the relational script she had begun to internalise. The following vignette illustrates how these procedural templates take shape and how quickly they become the organising grammar of the dyad.

Observation 15

Imogen was lying on her back on the play mat when I arrived, in a calm, alert state. Bernie sat beside her, talking softly and stroking her tummy. Imogen responded with smiles and animated arm and leg movements. Their interaction had a familiar rhythm: Bernie would speak or smile, and Imogen would answer with bodily excitement and widening eyes. The sequence had the feel of an established pattern, one that both partners seemed to recognise.

At one point, Bernie leaned over Imogen and said, "Where's that smile?" Imogen immediately responded with a broad grin, as though anticipating the familiar cue. Bernie laughed and repeated the phrase, and Imogen again smiled in synchrony. The exchange had a predictable structure: Bernie initiated, Imogen responded, and Bernie amplified the response. It was clear that Imogen had come to expect this pattern and was actively participating in its recreation.

Later, Bernie lifted Imogen into a sitting position. Imogen's face lit up, and she vocalised softly. Bernie echoed the sound, and Imogen repeated it with slightly more intensity. The back-and-forth had a playful, expectant quality, as though Imogen were testing how Bernie would respond. When Bernie briefly turned her attention to her older daughter, Imogen's expression changed; she became still, her gaze fixed on Bernie, waiting. As soon as Bernie returned her attention, Imogen resumed her vocalisations, and the rhythm was restored.

During a brief period of fussiness, Imogen arched her back and vocalised in protest. Bernie picked her up and held her close, rocking gently. Imogen settled quickly, then looked up at Bernie with a soft, open expression. The shift from dysregulation to calm seemed to rely on Bernie's predictable soothing pattern – another example of an interactional script that Imogen had come to expect.

Reflecting on the observation, what stood out was the emergence of procedural expectancies. Imogen appeared to recognise and anticipate Bernie's characteristic ways of initiating, soothing, and responding. Her smiles, vocalisations, and bodily movements were not random but seemed organised around these familiar sequences. She was beginning to use expressive behaviour instrumentally – to elicit a response, to test a pattern, to restore a rhythm.

This observation illustrates how early RIGs take shape. The dyad's repeated micro-exchanges were becoming internalised as procedural templates: "this is how we do things together". These templates guided Imogen's timing, her affective shifts, and her expectations of Bernie's availability. In adult psychotherapy, similar procedural patterns often emerge in the transference, where the patient anticipates the therapist's responses based on early relational scripts. The observation offers a vivid example of how such expectancies are formed long before language, through the choreography of everyday interaction.

Schore and the Psychobiology of Early Regulation

Schore's (1994) work converges with Stern's (1985) in emphasising the non-verbal, right-hemisphere-mediated processes through which affect is communicated and regulated. He argues that early caregiver–infant exchanges involve rapid, implicit psychobiological communication that facilitates the matching of internal states. Empathy, in this view, is best understood as a form of non-verbal attunement that supports the infant's developing capacity for self-regulation. When these processes fail, the infant's ability to regulate pre-symbolic affect is compromised, increasing vulnerability to later psychopathology.

Schore's (1994) integration of attachment research with neurobiology highlights the developmental roots of the emotion-regulation difficulties so often encountered in adult psychotherapy. Failures of early regulation leave the individual vulnerable to dysregulated states that may later manifest as dissociation, affect storms, or rigid defensive patterns. His work underscores the continuity between early relational processes and the implicit, procedural patterns that emerge in the therapeutic relationship.

From Infant Research to Adult Psychotherapy: The Procedural Past in the Consulting Room

The bridge from infant research to adult psychotherapy becomes clearest when we consider the role of implicit or procedural memory. Fonagy (1998) and the Boston Change Process Study Group have shown that much of what shapes adult relational life is encoded not as explicit narrative but as procedural knowledge – patterns of expectation, timing, and affective response that operate outside awareness. These patterns are enacted in the therapeutic relationship through tone, rhythm, pauses, and micro-shifts in affect.

Fonagy (1998) argues that the "schematic representations" described by attachment and object-relations theorists are best understood as procedural memories that adapt social behaviour to specific relational contexts. Patterns of attachment, therefore, are stored not as stories but as ways of relating. This perspective lends new significance to Ainsworth et al.'s (1978) strange situation procedure, which assesses the infant's procedural repertoire with a specific caregiver. In adults, attachment security is similarly inferred from the procedures used to create an attachment-related narrative.

Main's (1991) development of the Adult Attachment Interview provides compelling evidence for this view. She identified four parental states of mind with respect to attachment – secure/autonomous, dismissing, preoccupied, and unresolved – and demonstrated that these classifications predicted the infant's later attachment behaviour. Secure/autonomous parents showed coherent reflection on experience, whereas parents classified as Unresolved displayed lapses in reasoning and discourse when discussing trauma. Such lapses suggest dissociated, incompatible belief systems and "state shifts" in which the individual enters a compartmentalised, traumatic state of mind. These parental states were associated with disorganised attachment in the child.

Taken together, these findings show that each pattern of attachment organisation corresponds to a specific pattern of early caregiver–infant interaction and its behavioural sequelae. Van IJzendoorn's meta-analysis (van IJzendoorn, 1995) confirmed the predictive validity of the AAI, underscoring the value of a procedure-oriented psychodynamic approach. The significance of attachment research is examined in greater detail in Chapter 5.

Part III

Intersubjectivity and the Developmental Object in Adult Treatment

The intersubjective turn in psychoanalysis has brought infant research and adult psychotherapy into closer dialogue. Fonagy (1998), the Boston Change Process Study Group (Stern et al., 1998a, 1998b), Benjamin (1995), Hurry (1998), Tähkä (1993), and others converge on a shared insight: therapeutic change arises not primarily through interpretation but through the micro-processes of the relationship itself. These processes echo the early caregiver–infant exchanges that shape the developing mind.

Fonagy emphasises that the therapist becomes a new developmental object whose presence enables the patient to depart from entrenched relational procedures. The therapist's attunement, reliability, and capacity to mentalise the patient's experience creates a relational environment in which implicit patterns can be recognised, reorganised, and eventually symbolised. Stern et al.'s concepts of "now moments" and "moments of meeting" capture the immediacy of these encounters: brief, affectively charged events in which two subjectivities genuinely meet. When such moments are successfully negotiated, they open a space for new relational possibilities.

Benjamin (1995) adds that growth often occurs not through perfect empathy but through empathic failures that are survived. The analyst's capacity to withstand the patient's omnipotent destructive fantasies without retaliating allows the patient to recognise the analyst as a separate, usable other. This recognition marks a developmental shift, echoing the infant's dawning awareness of the caregiver as both connected and distinct.

Hurry (1998) similarly argues that developmental and therapeutic processes are inherently interactional. Patients who have suffered neglect or disappointment may struggle to trust a benign relationship and instead rely defensively on familiar but distorted internal working models. Yet alongside this defensive repetition lies an unconscious wish for change – a hope that the therapist will function as a developmental rather than a transferential object. In unconsciously asking the therapist to contradict transference expectations, the patient seeks an appropriate developmental object. This search may constitute the patient's real agenda and the foundation of a genuine, if largely unspoken, therapeutic alliance.

Tähkä's (1993) contribution is particularly pertinent here. He proposes that structural change arises from the patient's use of the analyst as a new developmental object – a position consistent with Benjamin's emphasis on the intertwining of interpersonal and intrapsychic processes. In a successful analysis, the analyst's fate as a developmental object mirrors what should have occurred with the original caregivers: a gradual, relative relinquishment of the analyst as both self-ideal and ideal love object.

Dyadic Systems, Corrective Experience, and the Choreography of Change

Lachmann and Beebe (1990) offer a complementary model of transference grounded in dyadic systems theory. They integrate the patient's enduring internal structures with the real-time interactional patterns emerging in the analytic dyad. In their view, interpersonal and intrapsychic sources operate concurrently throughout treatment. The therapist's task is to recognise the procedural patterns enacted in the relationship and to offer new relational experiences that challenge and expand the patient's repertoire.

The concept of a corrective emotional experience, first articulated by Alexander and French (1946), is reframed in this context. Rather than a single dramatic event, corrective experience becomes a series of micro--regulatory exchanges in which the therapist responds differently from the original caregivers. These differences – subtle, repeated, and cumulative – gradually reshape the patient's procedural expectations.

Kantrowitz's (1995) long-term follow-up study underscores the importance of the patient–analyst match. She found that the quality of fit between patient and analyst was the primary factor associated with successful outcome. Hurry argues that such matching is especially crucial for the spontaneous developmental aspects of treatment. Yet she also notes the countertransferential risks inherent in developmental work: the analyst may unconsciously use the patient to gratify narcissistic needs, relieve guilt, or meet their own infantile longings. Such risks require ongoing self-reflective monitoring of the countertransference.

Affect, Regulation, and the Therapist's Embodied Mind

Schore's contribution brings the discussion back to the psychobiological foundations of relational life. He argues that developmental research is directly relevant to adult psychotherapy because both rely on interactive, emotion-regulating mechanisms. In treating emotional dysregulation rooted in failures of early affective development, the therapist must match the patient's developmental level. Non-verbal internal working models of insecure attachment should be a central focus of treatment.

Interactive regulation of affect is, in Schore's view, a fundamental mechanism of both psychobiological development and therapeutic change. The therapeutic alliance becomes a mutually regulating system in which the patient's attachment capacities interact with the therapist's facilitating behaviours. For this process to succeed, the patient must experience the therapist as being in a state of "vitalising attunement".

Schore conceptualises defence mechanisms as "emotion regulation strategies" designed to avoid intolerable affect and prevent entry into "dreaded states" charged with intense negative emotion. His model emphasises primitive affects – shame, disgust, elation, excitement, terror, rage – rather than guilt and anxiety. The therapeutic task is to recognise and identify dissociated affects that have never been developmentally regulated or internally represented. This requires attention to discrete, automatic, facially and prosodically expressed affects, and to the intensity, duration, and lability of emotional states. Such work demands moment-to-moment tracking of subtle and dramatic shifts in affect and mood. Schore argues that this level of psychobiological attunement requires the therapist to use their visceral–somatic countertransference responses to the patient's internal state.

An Integrative Perspective: The Co-creation of Mind

Across these models, early development emerges as a fundamentally intersubjective process in which states of consciousness – affective, attentional, and intentional – are co-created within the dyad. A later observation, made when the infant was six and a half months old, offered a striking example of this co-creation of experience. By this stage, the infant was beginning to use the caregiver's mind as a reference point, seeking confirmation, reassurance, and meaning through subtle acts of looking and turning. What emerged was a small but unmistakable moment of shared intentionality – a glimpse of the infant's growing capacity to negotiate separation, explore the environment, and return to the caregiver for emotional anchoring. The following vignette illustrates how intersubjectivity takes shape in these early exchanges.

Observation 16

Imogen was lying on her back on the play mat when I arrived, in a calm, alert state. Bernie sat beside her, talking softly and stroking her tummy. Imogen responded with smiles and animated movements. After a few minutes, Bernie lifted her into a sitting position. Imogen's face lit up, and she vocalised softly. Bernie echoed the sound, and Imogen repeated it with slightly more intensity. Their exchange had a familiar rhythm, with each partner anticipating the other's next move.

When Bernie briefly turned her attention to her older daughter, Imogen's expression changed. She became still, her gaze fixed on Bernie, waiting. As soon as Bernie returned her attention, Imogen resumed her vocalisations, and the rhythm was restored. The shift was subtle but immediate, revealing how closely Imogen monitored Bernie's availability.

Later, Bernie handed Imogen to me while she prepared a bottle. As I held her, I became aware of a sudden uncertainty about how close to be. Imogen looked at me briefly, then turned away, her body slightly stiffening. I felt a corresponding tension in myself – a sense of being too intrusive if I moved closer, too distant if I held back. The moment had a delicate, finely balanced quality, as though Imogen were signalling that she needed space while still wanting some degree of connection.

I adjusted my position, softening my gaze and loosening my hold. Imogen's body relaxed almost immediately. She turned back toward me, her expression more open, and made a soft vocalisation. I responded quietly, matching her tone. A gentle rhythm developed: she would look at me, then look away; I would follow her lead, modulating my presence in response to her cues. The interaction felt like a negotiation of proximity and distance, with Imogen guiding the process through subtle shifts in gaze and posture.

At one point, Imogen's gaze drifted past me, and her expression took on a faraway quality. My own internal state shifted in response; I felt calmer, more spacious, as though drawn into her reflective mood. When she returned her gaze to me, I matched her softened expression with a quiet smile. The moment felt attuned and mutually regulating.

When Bernie returned and took Imogen in her arms, the infant immediately nestled into her, her body softening further. The contrast highlighted how finely tuned Imogen was to the nuances of relational presence and how quickly she responded to changes in the interpersonal field.

Reflecting on the observation, what stood out was the degree to which my own internal experience mirrored Imogen's subtle cues. The oscillation between closeness and distance, and the uncertainty about how to position myself, offered a vivid example of how the observer's countertransference becomes an instrument for sensing the infant's unformulated experience. Imogen's shifts in gaze, posture, and affect guided the interaction, and my own embodied responses provided additional information about her regulatory needs.

In clinical terms, the vignette illustrates the delicate negotiation of proximity and distance that often emerges in adult psychotherapy, particularly with patients whose early experiences have made closeness both desired and anxiety-provoking. The therapist's capacity to tolerate uncertainty, to adjust their stance moment by moment, and to use their own internal responses as data is central to working with such dynamics. The observation offers a clear example of how these processes originate in early relational life and how they are enacted in the implicit domain of therapeutic interaction.

While the caregiver's responsiveness is crucial, the infant's own emerging self-regulatory capacities also play a central role. Maladaptive patterns of interaction, whether through misattunement, defensive exclusion of signals, or failures of containment, may become internalised as enduring relational configurations that shape later personality and clinical presentations.

Infant observation, when reframed as a stance of receptive attunement, trains the clinician to track these implicit processes as they emerge in the therapeutic relationship. The observer learns to tolerate ambiguity, to sense the patient's unformulated experience, and to recognise patterns of attunement and misattunement without rushing to explanation. This stance mirrors the clinician's position in adult psychotherapy, where therapeutic action often depends on the capacity to receive and metabolise implicit relational communication before interpretation becomes possible.

A later observation brought this home with particular force, not only through the infant's behaviour but through the impact the encounter had on me as observer. I found myself oscillating between feeling too close and too distant, struggling to locate the right relational stance – an experience that mirrored the infant's own shifting signals. The vignette that follows captures this delicate negotiation of proximity and distance and illustrates how the observer's countertransference becomes an essential instrument for sensing the infant's unformulated experience.

Observation 22

When I arrived, Imogen was sitting on the floor supported by cushions, in a calm and alert state. Bernie sat opposite her, talking softly and offering a toy. Imogen reached for it with deliberate movements, glancing up at Bernie as she did so. The sequence had a distinctly triadic quality: Imogen looked at the toy, then at Bernie, then back at the toy, as though checking Bernie's mind for confirmation. Bernie responded with an encouraging smile and a gentle "Yes ... that's it", and Imogen's movements became more confident.

A little later, Imogen dropped the toy and looked towards Bernie with a questioning expression. Bernie retrieved it and handed it back, and Imogen smiled broadly. The exchange had the feel of early social referencing: Imogen appeared to be using Bernie's reaction to organise her own experience, seeking reassurance and meaning through Bernie's face and tone.

When Bernie briefly turned to speak to her older daughter, Imogen's expression changed. She became still, her gaze fixed on Bernie, waiting for her attention to return. As soon as Bernie turned back, Imogen's face lit up, and she vocalised softly. Bernie echoed the sound, and Imogen repeated it with more intensity. The rhythm of their interaction resumed immediately, as though a circuit had been reconnected.

Later, Imogen leaned forward, reaching towards a brightly coloured object on the floor. She paused, looked back at Bernie, and then resumed her reach. Bernie nodded and said "Go on", in a warm tone. Imogen grasped the object and looked back at Bernie with a triumphant expression. The sequence was subtle but unmistakable: Imogen was using Bernie's mind as a guide, checking her emotional availability and drawing on her as a secure base from which to explore.

At one point, Imogen became momentarily unsettled. She frowned, vocalised in a low tone, and looked toward Bernie with a slightly distressed expression. Bernie responded by leaning in, softening her voice, and placing a hand gently on Imogen's back. Imogen's body relaxed almost immediately. She looked up at Bernie, then back at me, and smiled. The shift from uncertainty to calm seemed to depend on Bernie's attuned presence and the predictability of her soothing response.

Reflecting on the observation, what stood out was the emergence of early intersubjectivity. Imogen was no longer simply engaging in dyadic exchanges but was beginning to use Bernie's mind as a reference point – seeking confirmation, reassurance, and meaning through subtle acts of looking and turning. Her exploration of the environment was organised around Bernie's availability; when Bernie's attention shifted, Imogen paused, waited, and then resumed once the connection was restored.

In clinical terms, the vignette illustrates how the infant's developing sense of self is shaped within a relational matrix in which the caregiver's mind becomes a regulatory and interpretive resource. The early forms of social referencing and shared attention seen here are precursors to the capacity for mentalisation and to the patient's later use of the therapist as a developmental object. The observation offers a clear example of how intersubjective processes take shape in infancy and how they form the procedural foundations of later relational life.

Conclusion

The Continuity of Early and Later Relational Life

The observational vignettes included in this chapter make visible the micro-processes through which early relational life is organised – the rhythms of attunement, rupture, repair, expectancy, and shared attention. These same implicit procedures reappear in adult psychotherapy, where the clinician's capacity to sense and respond to such patterns becomes central to therapeutic action.

The continuity between infant observation and adult psychotherapy lies not in descriptive parallels but in the mode of attention each cultivates. Infant observation trains the observer to track micro-shifts in affect and behaviour, tolerate uncertainty, and sense unformulated experience without premature interpretation. This stance becomes the clinical sensibility: receptive, attuned, and capable of holding experience until meaning can be co-constructed.

The "good enough" caregiver–infant relationship becomes a prototype for therapeutic action. Both involve subtle, reciprocal processes of regulation, misattunement, and repair. Theoretical frameworks from systems theory, interactionism, phenomenology, and social constructivism underscore that observation is never neutral - the observer is part of the relational field.

For this reason, those undertaking infant observation must adopt a method consonant with contemporary developmental and relational models – one that recognises the procedural past as it emerges in the present moment of the therapeutic encounter. In this way, infant observation serves not only as a window into early development, but as foundational training in the clinician's capacity to receive, contain, and work with the implicit relational life of the patient.

The next chapter extends this developmental lens into the forensic domain, showing how early relational failures – particularly prolonged separation and misattunement – shape later aggression, dissociation, and moral development. When such procedural patterns are organised under conditions of chronic threat and misattunement, their later expression may take forms that are socially disturbing and clinically difficult to bear.

References

Ainsworth, M. D. S. (1982). Attachment: Retrospect and prospect. In C. M. Parkes & J. Stevenson-Hinde (eds), *The place of attachment in human behavior* (pp. 3–30). New York: Basic Books.

Ainsworth, M. D. S., Blehar, M. C., Waters, E. & Wall, S. (1978). *Patterns of attachment: A psychological study of the strange situation*. Hillsdale, NJ: Erlbaum.

Alexander, F. & French, T. M. (1946). *Psychoanalytic therapy: Principles and application*. New York: Ronald Press.

Beebe, B., Jaffe, J. & Lachmann, F. M. (1992). A dyadic systems view of communication. In N. Skolnick & S. Warshaw (eds), *Relational perspectives in psychoanalysis* (pp. 61–81). Hillsdale, NJ: Analytic Press.

Beebe, B., Jaffe, J., Feldstein, S., Mays, K. & Alson, D. (1985). Interpersonal timing: The application of an adult dialogue model to mother–infant vocal and kinesic interactions. In T. M. Field & N. A. Fox (eds), *Social perception in infants* (pp. 217–247). Norwood, NJ: Ablex.

Benjamin, J. (1995). *Like subjects, love objects: Essays on recognition and sexual difference*. New Haven, CT: Yale University Press.

Bion, W. R. (1984). *Elements of psychoanalysis*. London: Karnac Books.

Bollas, C. (1987). *The shadow of the object: Psychoanalysis of the unthought known*. London: Free Association Books.

Bowlby, J. (1998). *Attachment and loss, vol. 3. Loss: Sadness and depression*. London: Pimlico.

Fairbairn, W. R. D. (1952). *Psychoanalytic studies of the personality*. London: Tavistock Publications.

Fonagy, P. (1998). An attachment theory approach to treatment of the difficult patient. *Bulletin of the Menninger Clinic*, 62(2), 147–169.

Fonagy, P. and Target, M. (1998). *Mentalization and the changing aims of child psychoanalysis*. London: Routledge.

Hurry, A. (1998). The developmental object in psychoanalysis. In A. Hurry (ed.), *Psychoanalysis and developmental therapy* (pp. 32–73). London: Karnac Books.

Jaffe, J., Beebe, B., Feldstein, S., Crown, C. & Jasnow, M. (2001). Rhythms of dialogue in infancy. *Monographs of the Society for Research in Child Development*, 66 (2), 1–132.

Kantrowitz, J. L. (1995). The patient's impact on the analyst. *Psychoanalytic Quarterly*, 64, 431–466.

Lachmann, F. M. & Beebe, B. (1990). On the origins of self- and object representations. *Psychoanalytic Psychology*, 7(1), 49–74.

Mahler, M. S., Pine, F. & Bergman, A. (1985). *The psychological birth of the human infant: Symbiosis and individuation*. London: Karnac Books.

Main, M. (1991). Metacognitive knowledge, metacognitive monitoring, and coherent vs. incoherent models of attachment. In C. M. Parkes, J. Stevenson-Hinde & P. Marris (eds), *Attachment across the life cycle* (pp. 127–159). London: Routledge.

Main, M. & Hesse, E. (1990). Parents' unresolved traumatic experiences are related to infant disorganized attachment status. In M. Greenberg, D. Cicchetti & E. Cummings (eds), *Attachment in the preschool years* (pp. 161–182). Chicago, IL: University of Chicago Press.

Main, M., Kaplan, N. & Cassidy, J. (1985). Security in infancy, childhood, and adulthood: A move to the level of representation. In I. Bretherton & E. Waters (eds), *Growing points in attachment: Theory and research* (pp. 66–104). Chicago, IL: University of Chicago Press.

Schore, A. N. (1994). *Affect regulation and the origin of the self: The neurobiology of emotional development*. Hillsdale, NJ: Lawrence Erlbaum Associates.

Stern, D. N. (1985). *The interpersonal world of the infant: A view from psychoanalysis and developmental psychology*. New York: Basic Books.

Stern, D. N., Sander, L. W., Nahum, J. P., Harrison, A. M., Lyons-Ruth, K., Morgan, A. C., Bruschweiler-Stern, N. & Tronick, E. Z. (1998a). Non-interpretive mechanisms in psychoanalytic therapy: The "something more" than interpretation. *International Journal of Psychoanalysis*, 79, 903–921.

Stern, D. N., Sander, L. W., Nahum, J. P., Harrison, A. M., Lyons-Ruth, K., Morgan, A. C., Bruschweiler-Stern, N. & Tronick, E. Z. (1998b). The process of therapeutic change involving implicit knowledge: Some implications of developmental observations for adult psychotherapy. *Infant Mental Health Journal*, 19(3), 300–308.

Tähkä, V. (1993). *Mind and its treatment: A psychoanalytic approach*. Madison, CT: International Universities Press.

Tronick, E. Z., Als, H., Adamson, L., Wise, S. & Brazelton, T. B. (1978). The infant's response to entrapment between contradictory messages in face-to-face interaction. *Journal of the American Academy of Child Psychiatry*, 17(1), 1–13.

Tyson, P. & Tyson, R. L. (1990). *Psychoanalytic theories of development: An integration*. New Haven, CT: Yale University Press.

van der Kolk, B. A. (1994). The body keeps the score. *Harvard Review of Psychiatry*, 1(5), 253–265.

van der Kolk, B. A. & Fisler, R. (1995). Dissociation and the fragmentary nature of traumatic memories. *Journal of Traumatic Stress*, 8(4), 505–525.

van IJzendoorn, M. H. (1995). Adult attachment representations, parental responsiveness, and infant attachment. *Psychological Bulletin*, 117(3), 387–403.

Winnicott, D. W. (1958). The capacity to be alone. *International Journal of Psychoanalysis*, 39, 416–420.

Winnicott, D. W. (1988). *Human nature*. London: Free Association Books.

Part II

Cumulative Trauma, Memory, and Intergenerational Transmission

Introduction to Part II

Part I examined how relational patterns are formed, Part II turns to what happens when those patterns are shaped by chronic relational failure. This section develops cumulative trauma as the book's central organising concept and explores the mechanisms through which traumatic relational experience becomes encoded in memory and transmitted across generations.

Cumulative trauma differs fundamentally from discrete traumatic events. It does not arise from dramatic rupture but from repetitive patterns of misattunement, failures of recognition, and absences of repair. It is the trauma of what should have happened but did not – of responses that were needed and unavailable, of affective states that could not be held or regulated. Because it unfolds within ordinary developmental contexts and often within ostensibly "good enough" caregiving, cumulative trauma frequently remains invisible and unnamed.

Despite its subtlety, its effects are far-reaching. Cumulative trauma shapes capacities for affect regulation, emotional recognition, trust in relationship, and the experience of agency. It is encoded primarily in procedural memory – not as discrete events that can be recalled, but as implicit patterns of expectation, defensive organisation, and relational engagement. These patterns are transmitted across generations through the quality of caregiver–child interaction, creating intergenerational cycles that operate largely outside conscious awareness.

The five chapters in this section approach cumulative trauma from complementary perspectives.

Chapter 4 opens with a clinical vignette drawn from forensic work with juvenile violence. Drawing on Bowlby's early thinking, it illustrates how attachment disruption and cumulative relational failure can be enacted through violence. The question "what has been stolen and by whom?" introduces the existential dimensions of cumulative trauma: compromised agency, failures of recognition, and the experience of something profoundly missing.

DOI: 10.4324/9781003789727-6

Chapter 5 provides the theoretical core of the volume. It defines cumulative trauma in depth, distinguishes it from discrete trauma and from ordinary developmental failure, and examines the mechanisms through which it forms and is transmitted. Integrating psychoanalytic theory, attachment research, and contemporary neuroscience, this chapter offers a comprehensive framework for understanding cumulative trauma's origins, manifestations, and persistence.

Chapter 6 focuses on memory systems and the encoding of traumatic experience. Distinguishing between implicit and explicit memory, and between procedural and declarative knowing, it explores how experiences that cannot be symbolised or narrated nonetheless shape subjectivity through dissociation, fragmentation, and somatic organisation. The therapeutic relationship is positioned as the site where such fragmented experience may gradually find integration.

Chapter 7 revisits Kleinian theory through the lens of cumulative trauma. It asks how internal object worlds develop under conditions of chronic relational failure, and how processes such as splitting, persecutory anxiety, and projective identification relate to failures of containment and recognition. Rather than reducing Klein to attachment theory or discarding her insights, this chapter places classical psychoanalysis in dialogue with contemporary trauma perspectives.

Chapter 8 examines power asymmetry as a central but under-theorised dimension of attachment and cumulative trauma. Experiences of authority, coercion, and misrecognition are shown to shape the developing self and to operate across both developmental and therapeutic relationships. This chapter prepares the ground for Part III's focus on enactment, ethics, boundaries, and the inherent power dynamics of the consulting room.

Taken together, these chapters establish that cumulative trauma is not exceptional but a common dimension of development; that its transmission operates procedurally, through implicit patterns of regulation and recognition rather than conscious intention; that traumatic experience may be encoded somatically and fragmentarily, resisting coherent narrative; and that power and context matter profoundly, with systemic factors such as racism, poverty, and social marginalisation shaping developmental risk without collapsing into parent-blaming or biological determinism.

These insights have significant clinical implications. If cumulative trauma is common rather than exceptional, presentations often understood as character pathology or treatment resistance may instead be recognised as adaptive responses to chronic relational failure. If transmission is procedural, therapeutic change requires attention to what happens between people, not only to explicit beliefs or conscious intention. And if memory systems are multiple, therapeutic work must engage enacted and embodied experience as well as narrative meaning.

Part II thus extends the developmental foundations established in Part I by examining how relational failure becomes structured into personality and carried forward across generations. It provides the conceptual framework for the clinical challenges explored in Part III, where these patterns emerge in enactment, boundary dilemmas, erotic transference, and work with patients whose core difficulties arise from cumulative relational trauma.

The question animating this section is: how does relational failure become encoded in memory, organised into personality, and transmitted across generations? Addressing this question is essential not only for theoretical clarity, but for clinical effectiveness. We cannot help our patients transform what we, ourselves, do not understand.

4 Stop Thief! But What Has Been Stolen and By Whom?

Commentary on a Paper by John Bowlby

Retrospective Reflection

This chapter was written at a time when my clinical and theoretical interests were increasingly shaped by the encounter between attachment theory and work within forensic and probation settings. Returning to it now, I am struck by how clearly Bowlby's early observations anticipated many of the concerns that have since come to be articulated under the rubric of cumulative relational trauma, even though such language was not available to him at the time. This later articulation of cumulative trauma, including its developmental mechanisms and intergenerational transmission, is developed in detail in Chapter 5.

Bowlby's insistence on the centrality of real relational experience, prolonged separation, and emotional deprivation challenged dominant psychoanalytic assumptions about the primacy of intrapsychic phantasy. In doing so, it opened a pathway for thinking about how chronic failures of care shape affect regulation, moral development, and the capacity for relatedness. From the perspective developed later in this volume, these processes can be understood as cumulative and developmental in nature, unfolding over time through repeated relational disruption rather than discrete traumatic events.

The clinical material discussed here, drawn from work with violent young men, illustrates how early attachment disturbance may be carried forward into later enactments of aggression and disorganisation. Read in the context of subsequent chapters, this material can also be understood as prefiguring later discussions of dissociation, intergenerational transmission, and the restoration of agency within relationship. The chapter therefore functions as a bridge between foundational attachment theory and the more explicitly relational and clinical focus that follows.

Introduction

John Bowlby's contribution to psychoanalytic thinking represented a decisive shift in emphasis from intrapsychic phantasy to the lived realities of

DOI: 10.4324/9781003789727-7

early relational experience. His work foregrounded the developmental consequences of prolonged separation, emotional deprivation, and loss, insisting that such experiences exert a shaping influence on personality, behaviour, and the capacity for moral relatedness.

Bowlby's position was controversial in its time, not least because it challenged prevailing assumptions about the origins of disturbance. Rather than locating pathology primarily in unconscious conflict, he drew attention to the cumulative impact of disrupted attachment relationships and the absence of reliable caregiving. From a contemporary perspective, this can be understood as an early articulation of what is now conceptualised as cumulative relational trauma: the gradual shaping of internal experience through repeated failures of protection, attunement, and repair. The concept of cumulative trauma is developed more fully in Chapter 5.

This chapter revisits Bowlby's thinking through the lens of clinical work with young people involved in violent and antisocial behaviour. In doing so, it explores how early attachment disturbance may find expression in aggression, dissociation, and difficulties with affect regulation. The discussion is concerned less with retrospective explanation than with understanding how such patterns emerge developmentally and how they might be addressed within relational contexts of care and treatment. Although this paper predates the formal articulation of attachment theory, many of the ideas that later became central were already present.

The Child's Phenomenological Experience

In exploring the child's phenomenological experience, Bowlby (1944) paid especial attention to the emotional atmosphere in the home. Instead of privileging unconscious phantasy, he stressed the significance of the child's real-life experiences and emotional relationships, arguing that these factors vitally influence the development of the child's character. He implicated parents' conscious and unconscious attitude towards their child, noting that this was often marked by ambivalence, rejection, and unacknowledged hatred and hostility. But he gave most weight to the child's prolonged separation from the mother, viewing this as the cause of "appalling damage" because it shattered the "emotional bonds which usually unite mother and child" (Bowlby, 1944, p. 112). When eventually reunited, the child felt like a "lost soul" and the mother as though she had "lost her child" (p. 112).

Bowlby points out how lightly early separations were treated by most workers in the field of juvenile delinquency. He advocates adopting a position of active inquiry into emotional traumas, stating "My experience has shown me again and again that if these factors are not looked for, they are not found" (Bowlby, 1944, p. 20). He criticised the prevailing attitude among professionals dealing with adult offenders for failing to take into account the early environment and current circumstances of the person in understanding their criminal behaviour.

Affectionless Characters

Of the forty-four children interviewed by Bowlby, fourteen were diagnosed as "affectionless characters". This section constitutes the heart of the paper. In addition to stealing and truanting, many of these children were aggressive and bullying. In respect of some, Bowlby (1944) formed the impression that "they might easily develop into desperate and dangerous criminals" (p. 38). While Bowlby considers that mothers have greater influence than fathers in their children's early years, in some of the cases studied he concluded that the father's malign influence was of outstanding importance in contributing to the child's unfavourable character development.

In the majority of cases, however, he found a high degree of association between the affectionless children and prolonged mother–child separation. These children were distinguished from their peers by being isolated, emotionally indifferent, and unresponsive in their personal relationships. Regardless of the real qualities of the mother, the child who has experienced a prolonged separation tends to distort their perceptions, seeing her as a faithless, malicious, and hateful person, and himself as a bad, unlovable object.

As Bowlby (1944) discovered, the characteristic avoidance and indifference of affectionless children was a form of self-protection against the risk of their ever again experiencing feelings of disappointment, rage, and longing for the lost or unavailable person. However, he noted that "behind the mask of indifference is bottomless misery, and behind the apparent callousness despair" (p. 39). Stealing, however unconsciously motivated, was a way of fulfilling hopes for "libidinal satisfaction", in that the objects stolen were felt to be the symbolic equivalent of the mother's love. But, as Bowlby notes, the act of stealing was also aggressive, being motivated by the deprived child's intention to inflict suffering on the other in equal measure to the suffering that had been inflicted on him. The role of power, misrecognition, and asymmetry in shaping such aggressive enactments is examined more explicitly in Chapter 8.

Bowlby's contribution to the field of juvenile delinquency gradually waned in the years following World War II, but his interest in the effects on children of real-life events continued apace with a research focus on separation and loss. Attachment theory has been in a continuous process of development and refinement, a process informed by a wealth of empirical studies.

Later Years

Some forty years after the publication of the study of forty-four thieves, Bowlby wrote a paper titled "Violence in the Family as a Disorder of the Attachment and Caregiving Systems" (Bowlby, 1984). He notes how "appallingly slow" psychoanalysts and psychotherapists have been in appreciating the prevalence and far-reaching consequences of violent behaviour between family members. In reflecting on his decision at the start of his professional working life to study separation and loss, rather than violence and abuse, he points to the fact that it had been unfashionable in psychoanalytic circles to attribute psychopathology to real-life experiences ever since Freud's (1897) partial repudiation of his seduction theory. Consequently, the adverse behaviour of parents towards their children had become a "taboo subject".

This explanation may account for the under-emphasis in the forty-four thieves study of childhood physical abuse and the curious absence of any mention of sexual abuse and concomitant states of dissociation, despite there being clear indications that such abuse had occurred in some cases. From a contemporary standpoint, these omissions are striking. These factors may be seen in case no. 27, Betty I., who was referred to the clinic when aged 5 years and 7 months. Betty had had a series of foster-homes since the age of seven months and had then spent a year at a convent school before being reunited with her mother and stepfather when five years old. Bowlby (1944) comments that Betty often "appeared to be walking along in a dream", adding that "Her tendency to be dreamy, to mix with undesirables and to have over-developed sexual interests were also striking" (p 40). The stepfather was said to be "particularly worried by her sexual interests, which seemed to be very active even for this age" (p. 40).

From the vantage point of our knowledge today, Betty's precocious sexual behaviour and dissociated state would suggest the distinct possibility that she had been sexually abused. Thus, although Bowlby advocated inquiring into the child's emotional traumas, his inquiries would seem to have been circumscribed in some degree by the taboos operating in the 1930s. The clinical implications of dissociative and fragmented states are taken up further in Chapter 12.

That said, his emphasis on the child's environment and real-life experiences was, in many respects, ground-breaking. He was particularly sensitive to the plight of the young child. The poignant stories he tells of these children suggest that they, themselves, had been the victims of a theft, and that what had been stolen from them was their very childhoods. We have John Bowlby to thank for helping us recognise the severe damage done to children by a cavalier disregard of their urgent need to feel safely and securely attached to a primary caregiver.

But what, we may ask, has attachment theory and research contributed to a contemporary understanding of criminal behaviour? Bowlby's original focus on separation, loss, and trauma has been refined and elaborated in the light of findings relating to disorganised attachment, the intergenerational transmission of trauma, affect regulation, and mentalisation. Despite the shift away from forensic issues, I found the ongoing work of Bowlby and his collaborators of particular help in understanding the clinical issues that underlie stalking and violent behaviour, in assessing the risk of dangerousness, and in working therapeutically with offenders who had committed serious crimes (Renn, 2003, 2006).

The relevance of these early insights becomes particularly evident when considered alongside contemporary clinical work with individuals whose developmental histories bear the imprint of similar relational disruptions.

Case Assessment: Andrew and Peter

The following case assessment of two brothers, Andrew and Peter, undertaken when I worked as a probation officer, illustrates salient theoretical points and the way in which loss, abuse, and trauma in early life are implicated in setting the child on a developmental pathway that may culminate in violent behaviour in later life. The exploration of the brothers' phenomenological experience remains true to Bowlby's exhortation in his forty-four thieves' paper, namely that the person's early formative experiences and current circumstances should be taken into account in understanding their offending behaviour.

Andrew had been living at the home of two drug-using friends, Colin and Mary, for about a year. His relationships with them deteriorated because of his feeling excluded and rejected. He and Mary occasionally had sex, but she decided to stay in the relationship with Colin. When Colin discovered what had been going on, he told Andrew to leave their home. Andrew responded in a rage, attacking Colin with his bare fists and beating him so seriously about the head that he died of his injuries some weeks later. Andrew, who was 31 at that point and also misusing drugs, was arrested and charged with murder.

Andrew is the second of four children, having a brother, Peter, who is two years older, and two younger half siblings. His mother had immigrated to Britain from the Caribbean when she was 17. Andrew has no memory of his biological father, who deserted the family when he was just 18 months old, leaving the mother to cope as best she could with little social or emotional support in a new country. Shortly after this, she sent the two brothers to Barbados to be raised by her parents. Some five years later, when she had established herself in a career and a new relationship, she arranged for the children to be returned to her. Andrew was then aged 7 and Peter was 9.

I had worked briefly with Peter some five years previously to meeting Andrew. Both he and Andrew told me that they had developed a close, loving relationship with their grandmother during their five-year stay in Barbados and had felt intense distress at having to leave her to return to England. This transition was particularly fraught because of the mother's routine emotional and physical abuse of her two young sons on their reunion.

Peter responded to this traumatic situation by manifesting emotional and behavioural problems at home and at his state school, where he was bullied and subjected to racist taunts, a situation not helped by his being separated from Andrew, who was educated at a different school. Peter became confused, withdrawn and socially isolated. He took to carrying a knife because he feared for his personal safety. At the age of 12, he began to refuse to attend school and was referred to a child psychologist. He refused to talk with her and so the therapy was discontinued. In his teens he developed a serious drink problem and was soon appearing before the courts. Peter's relationships with women were short-lived and often violent. He has numerous criminal convictions for assaulting his female partners, which have resulted in his being imprisoned on several occasions.

Andrew's distress was less evident than Peter's at the early stage of his development. He attended a private day school and was socially outgoing and popular with his peers. He applied himself to his scholastic studies and later attained a vocational qualification which helped him to remain in full time employment in the building industry. He turned to religion for solace in his teenage years and developed a good relationship with his stepfather, who he saw as protecting him from the worst excesses of his mother's violence and emotional abuse.

When Andrew was 19, he entered into his first serious intimate relationship with a woman. Some six years later, when he was 25, she ended the relationship. Although on the surface Andrew seemed unaffected by the loss, it soon became apparent that he was not coping with this stressful situation and that his life was falling apart. He resorted to alcohol and crack cocaine, heavily misusing both substances, and he emulated Peter by acting out in a sexually promiscuous way, fathering several children.

Andrew also felt the loss of his biological father keenly at that time and made strenuous efforts to trace him but without success. He became increasingly depressed and twice attempted suicide - by overdosing on paracetamol and by hanging himself, which led to brief admissions onto a psychiatric ward. However, the psychiatric assessments concluded that he was not suffering from a mental illness at that time, nor, indeed, five years later when he was again psychiatrically assessed prior to being sentenced for killing Colin.

From an attachment theory perspective, I see the roots of Andrew's and Peter's violence as residing in their unresolved traumatic experience of separation, loss, and abuse within a disorganised caregiving-attachment system. Despite the early loss of the father and separation from the mother, had the boys received appropriate help to securely re-attach to their mother, and thus to use her as a secure base to mourn the separation from the grandmother, their development may well have taken a different pathway. As it was, their sadness, fear and distress were cruelly dealt with and they were forced to adapt to a harsh reality and alien culture as best they could.

This fraught situation was further complicated by their experience of the mother as being not only powerful, dominant, and abusive, but also loving, caring and concerned that they should make a success of their lives. Thus, Andrew and Peter both loved her and feared and hated her. These ambivalent, conflicting feelings led to the development of a multiple, incompatible internal working model and to a concomitant disorganised pattern of attachment. As a consequence, their capacity to regulate negative feeling states and reflect on and organise traumatic experience was seriously compromised. Peter, in particular, displayed a pronounced tendency to react violently to even relatively insignificant personal slights, losses, and rejections. Such minor injuries to the sense of self seemed to activate the original separation trauma, together with unintegrated affective states of shame and rage associated with racism and physical and emotional abuse, and thus to elicit a response that was disproportionate to the current mortification.

Moreover, because of persisting states of insecurity and lack of trust, neither Andrew nor Peter was able to enter into a committed, emotionally mature relationship. It would seem that the prospect of becoming attached to another person elicited expectations that oscillated between fear of engulfment and fear of abandonment, as expressed in their respective catastrophic narratives. As a result, emotionally meaningful relationships were generally avoided and intimacy was defended against.

Andrew's affective reaction to rejection and abandonment by Colin and Mary could not be contained and processed but was instead acted out in a most violent fashion. In attachment terms, this situation re-traumatised Andrew, activating an archaic disorganised internal working model full of rage, shame, and hate. To what extent the legacy of slavery was also implicated, in terms of the intergenerational transmission of trauma and the impact this had on the parenting practices to which Andrew and Peter were subjected, are, I think, pertinent questions. Such actions can be understood as relational enactments in which unintegrated affect and early attachment trauma are lived out in the present, a process examined clinically in Chapter 10.

Andrew pleaded not guilty to murder but guilty to manslaughter. His plea was accepted by the prosecution and he was sentenced to six years' imprisonment. Following his release from prison on parole licence we worked on the clinical issues outlined above, as well as on intense feelings of guilt and shame, symptoms of post-traumatic stress deriving from having killed his friend, heroin addiction, and relationship difficulties with his current romantic partner.

We also explored why Andrew's mother had parented him as she had, setting this in the context of what we knew about her own early attachment history, her experience of separation and loss from home and loved ones in adolescence, and of abandonment by Andrew's father shortly after he was born. By means of this process, Andrew came to recognise and reflect on his mother's formative experiences and subjectivity, thereby organising and integrating the traumatising aspects of his relationship with her. This, in turn, helped us to understand the ways in which the internalised relational patterns with his mother were being externalised and destructively repeated in the relationship with his current partner. As we will explore further in

Chapter 5, the mother's experience of cultural dislocation can be understood not only in psychosocial terms but also through an epigenetic lens, shaping the relational environment into which Andrew and Peter were born.

Although Peter had not re-offended since my brief intervention with him five years ago, he remained a deeply unhappy and depressed man who was dependent on alcohol and whose relationships were in a perpetual state of conflict. He had not felt ready to fully engage in working with me on his difficulties in living when we had first met. This may partly have been because of my position as an authority figure and representative of the dominant white culture. However, he attended a session unannounced with his brother to ask if I could arrange for him to receive help with his problems. Both he and Andrew spoke of their intention to make a renewed effort to find their father and maintain contact with their own children.

Conclusion

From a developmental perspective, the behaviours described in this chapter can be understood as the downstream effects of early attachment disruption and prolonged emotional deprivation. Bowlby's work reminds us that violence and antisocial behaviour do not arise in a vacuum, nor can they be adequately understood through actuarial or decontextualised models of risk. Rather, they reflect attempts to manage overwhelming affect, threat, and loss in the absence of reliable relational containment.

Read in the context of the chapters that follow, this material underscores the importance of attending to cumulative relational trauma and its impact on the organisation of the self. It also anticipates later discussions of enactment, dissociation, and the therapeutic task of restoring agency and recognition within relationships. Bowlby's legacy, viewed in this way, lies not only in his theoretical contributions, but in his insistence that emotional suffering must be understood within the fabric of lived human relationships. What remains to be understood is how such relational disruptions accumulate over time and transmit across generations – a question that requires a different level of conceptual integration. Chapter 5 addresses this question directly.

Acknowledgement

This chapter was originally published as Renn (2007). It is reproduced with the kind permission of Karnac Books Limited.

References

Bowlby, J. (1944). Forty-four juvenile thieves: Their characters and home life. *International Journal of Psychoanalysis*, 25, 1–57, 207–228.

Bowlby, J. (1984). Violence in the family as a disorder of the attachment and caregiving systems. *American Journal of Psychoanalysis*, 44, 9–27.

Freud, S. (1897). Letter to Wilhelm Fliess, 21 September 1897. In J. M. Masson (ed.), *The complete letters of Sigmund Freud to Wilhelm Fliess, 1887–1904* (pp. 264–267). Cambridge, MA: Harvard University Press.

Renn, P. (2003). The link between childhood trauma and later violent offending: The application of attachment theory in a probation setting. In F. Pfäfflin & G. Adshead (eds), *A matter of security: The application of attachment theory to forensic psychiatry and psychotherapy* (pp. 109–144). London: Jessica Kingsley Publishers.

Renn, P. (2006). Attachment, trauma and violence: Understanding destructiveness from an attachment theory perspective. In C. Harding (ed.), *Aggression and destructiveness: Psychoanalytic perspectives* (pp. 57–78). London: Routledge.

Renn, P. (2007). Stop thief! But what has been stolen and by whom? Discussion of paper by John Bowlby. *Attachment: New Directions in Psychotherapy and Relational Psychoanalysis*, 1(1), 71–77.

5 The Concept of Cumulative Relational Trauma and the Processes of Intergenerational Transmission

Retrospective Reflection

This chapter represents a significant re-articulation of ideas that have been central to my work for many years. Although earlier versions of my thinking on cumulative trauma appeared in previous publications, the present chapter is not a simple revision but a substantial re-conceptualisation shaped by developments in relational psychoanalysis, attachment research, neurobiology, and epigenetics. Writing it for this volume has allowed me to integrate strands of theory that had previously remained adjacent: the procedural nature of early relational experience, the intergenerational transmission of trauma, the cultural and systemic contexts in which caregiving unfolds, and the neurobiological pathways through which stress and misattunement become embodied.

What has become increasingly clear to me over time is that cumulative relational trauma cannot be understood solely within a psychological or interpersonal frame. The last decade of research has illuminated how chronic misattunement, systemic oppression, and environmental stressors shape the developing stress-response system at molecular, neural, and relational levels. This expanded perspective has deepened my appreciation of cumulative trauma as a multi-layered process – simultaneously biological, psychological, cultural, and intergenerational.

In the architecture of this volume, the chapter now serves as a conceptual anchor. It consolidates the developmental foundations laid out earlier in the book and provides the theoretical scaffolding for the clinical material that follows. By situating cumulative trauma within a relational-neurodevelopmental framework, it prepares the reader for the later chapters on enactment, sexuality, violence, and severe disturbance, where these same processes become vividly alive in the therapeutic relationship. In this sense, the chapter reflects both continuity and evolution in my thinking: the core ideas remain, but they are now held within a broader, more integrated understanding of how trauma is formed, transmitted, and transformed. The integrative perspective that frames this chapter is introduced in Chapter 1, where the developmental, relational, and clinical strands brought together here are first outlined.

DOI: 10.4324/9781003789727-8

Introduction

Building on the integrative perspective outlined in the retrospective reflection above, this chapter offers a contemporary account of cumulative relational trauma[1] as a developmental, neurobiological, and intergenerational process. While the concept has deep roots in psychoanalytic and attachment theory, recent advances in neuroscience, epigenetics, and cultural studies allow for a more comprehensive understanding of how subtle relational disruptions become embedded in the child's implicit systems of regulation and meaning. My aim here is to articulate a framework that links these diverse strands of research, clarifying how early relational patterns are encoded, transmitted, and later enacted in clinical work. In doing so, the chapter provides the theoretical foundation for the clinical material that follows in this volume, where these processes become vividly alive in therapeutic relationships.

Cumulative relational trauma refers to the developmental impact of repeated relational disruptions – misattunement, inconsistent caregiving, and unresolved affective ruptures – whose effects may be profound, despite the absence of overt traumatic events. Far from being rare, these subtle yet chronic experiences shape the child's emerging regulatory capacities, implicit memory systems, and internal working models of self and other. Where the shortened term *cumulative trauma* is used in this volume, it refers to this relationally organised process, rather than to discrete traumatic events.

Findings from attachment research illustrate how cumulative trauma becomes embedded in the child's implicit relational system long before explicit memory is available. Implicit memory, then, is predominant in early life, and infants encode relational patterns in procedural, nonverbal systems. These systems or mental models shape later attachment states of mind, affect regulation, and the expectations we have of others. The origins of these implicit relational systems, and their observation in early caregiver–infant interaction, are explored in detail in Chapter 3.

While the research informing these concepts derives largely from infant-caregiver studies, these same procedural patterns manifest in the transference, in intimate relationships, and in the characteristic ways patients manage affect and connection. Thus, this developmental framework is essential for understanding and treating child, adolescent, and adult patients.

Cumulative trauma differs from chronic trauma in that the former may arise even in otherwise "good enough" families in which overt trauma is completely absent. There is a danger of privileging so-called "big T" trauma over cumulative, micro relational trauma, thereby failing to identify the developmental harm consequent on this more subtle form of trauma. I examine the processes by which parents transmit attachment states, fears, and unresolved trauma. These processes occur largely outside conscious awareness through repetitive behaviour, tone of voice, gaze, posture, and affect. Such subtle behaviours often reemerge in the transference, offering clinicians a window into parents' early attachment patterns and procedural forms of relating that otherwise remain inaccessible.

The framework I employ in examining these processes is mainly informed by an integrative psychosocial perspective, as set out in a previous publication (Renn, 2012). This reflects the fact that I am a relational psychoanalytic psychotherapist. However, I acknowledge that a psychological model frequently overlooks or minimises biological contributions informed by a medical model. Moreover, the emphasis on a psychosocial model risks making parents feel blamed for their children's various difficulties in living. Conversely, a medical model risks seeing relational factors as innate defects.

Thus, there is a tension between these different explanatory paradigms in exploring the same phenomena. Indeed, it may be argued that there is a political dimension to diagnosis, with psychiatrists and paediatricians having moved away from psychological theories that seemed to blame parents. Indeed, twin studies are often held up as the gold standard in behavioural genetics, being seen as providing robust evidence of genetic explanations for conditions such as autism. However, as Boomsma et al. (2002) and Polderman et al. (2015) argue, such studies have a number of fundamental methodological limitations.

Universal versus Cultural Dimensions to Cumulative Trauma

A parallel consideration concerns the relationship between universal and culturally specific dimensions of attachment and trauma. While the fundamental mechanisms of attachment formation and intergenerational transmission described in this chapter appear to operate across cultural contexts, the specific caregiving behaviours through which attunement is expressed and received vary significantly across cultures. Comprehensive cross-cultural research by van IJzendoorn and Sagi (1999) demonstrates that secure, insecure, and disorganized attachment patterns are identifiable across diverse societies worldwide. However, the distribution of these patterns, the normative expectations surrounding separation and autonomy, and the specific behaviours that constitute sensitive responsiveness differ meaningfully across cultural contexts.

This has direct implications for identifying cumulative trauma, in that what constitutes chronic misattunement must be understood within cultural frameworks of normative caregiving. Physical proximity that signals intrusive overinvolvement in one cultural context may represent normative attunement in another; conversely, parenting that fosters early independence in Western middle-class families might feel like abandonment in cultures prioritising interdependence. Throughout this chapter, when discussing interactive regulation, affect-mirroring, and reflective functioning, readers should therefore consider how these universal processes take culturally specific forms.

Crucially, clinicians should also recognise how systemic factors, such as racism, poverty, and cultural dislocation, operate as environmental stressors with epigenetic consequences. As discussed below, chronic exposure to systemic oppression and social marginalisation triggers neurobiological changes in stress-response systems that may compromise parents' capacity for consistent attunement, despite their best intentions and efforts (Meaney, 2010; Szyf & Bick, 2013). Parents navigating multiple cultural frameworks, subjected to discrimination, or coping with the intergenerational effects of historical trauma carry burdens that are simultaneously psychological, neurobiological, and social.

These, then, are not individual deficits but adaptive responses to overwhelming and unjust environmental conditions. The challenge for clinicians is to distinguish between culturally normative variations in caregiving patterns and genuine disruptions in attunement within any given cultural context, while simultaneously recognising how systemic oppression creates conditions in which cumulative trauma becomes more likely to develop and be transmitted across generations.

An Emerging Consensus and Epigenetic Considerations

Despite some entrenched positions, there are signs of an emerging consensus between these different perspectives, a consensus that views conditions such as ADHD and autism as neither simply brain disorders nor simply relational wounds, but rather as neurodevelopmental conditions expressed within relational, social, and cultural contexts (Bullmore, 2018, 2024). Such contextualisation recognises that parents themselves are embedded in stressful situations, have their own trauma histories, and are subjected to various societal pressures.

A growing body of epigenetic research demonstrates how early relational stress interacts with gene expression and stress-response systems (Meaney, 2010; Szyf & Bick, 2013). Specifically, Meaney found that variations in early maternal caregiving in rats alter the epigenetic regulation of the glucocorticoid receptor (GR) gene in the hippocampus, a key moderator of the stress response. While epigenetic modulation may *indirectly* shape a child's threshold for stress and vulnerability to parental misattunement, thereby amplifying the effects of cumulative trauma, such changes do not *directly* encode traumatic memories. DNA methylation is a primary biological mechanism by which environmental factors, such as nutrition and stress, influence gene activity (Heijmans, et al. 2008; Yehuda, et al. 2016).

These epigenetic findings, then, have profound implications for understanding cumulative trauma within broader social contexts. Chronic exposure to systemic stressors – racism, poverty, immigration trauma, cultural dislocation – constitutes precisely the kind of early stressful environment that Meaney (2010) and Szyf and Bick (2013) respectively identify as triggering epigenetic changes in stress-response systems.

A parent living under precarious economic conditions, experiencing daily discrimination, or coping with the ongoing effects of forced migration is not merely psychologically stressed but epigenetically impacted in ways that may compromise regulatory capacity and attunement. The chronic activation of stress response systems under conditions of systemic oppression alters the very neurobiological substrate available for caregiving.

Moreover, these epigenetic effects may themselves be transmitted intergenerationally, such that historical trauma, including slavery, genocide, and colonisation, continue to shape stress response systems and attachment neurobiology across generations. Research on Holocaust survivors and their descendants, for example, demonstrates detectable epigenetic signatures of trauma transmission (Yehuda et al. 2016).

This perspective reveals systemic oppression not merely as a social issue separate and distinct from biology, but as an environmental factor with direct neurobiological consequences that increase vulnerability to cumulative trauma. Recognising racism, poverty, and cultural trauma as epigenetic factors emphasises that working with cumulative trauma requires attention not only to individual therapeutic processes, but also to the societal conditions that shape biological vulnerability and resilience across generations.

From a public health perspective, and reflecting the concern of many parents, the emphasis is on the erosion of attention in a digital age, resulting in the quiet displacement of emotional presence in early life. When the parent–child bond is diluted by the constant distraction of, not to say addiction to, digital devices, it is not merely time together that is lost, but the subtle, reciprocal dance through which trust, security, and empathy are first learned (Princess of Wales and Waldinger, 2025).

Developmental epigenetics indicate that such relational impoverishment may reach beyond behaviour or feeling, shaping the very biological scripts that govern stress, attachment, and neural growth. In this sense, the concern here evokes an epigenetic vision of human development – one in which love and attention are not just psychological nutrients, but molecular ones as well.

In this context, Zuckerman's (1998) work on molecular analysis helps explain how psychological phenomena arise from biological substrates. Such holistic, integrative models connect biology, psychology, and lived experience. His biologically grounded but non-deterministic model seeks to illustrate how personality emerges from the dynamic interplay between inherited neurochemical disposition and environmental experience.

Zuckerman argues that variations in such genetic data influence arousal thresholds, stress responsivity, and reward sensitivity, which in turn shape enduring behavioural tendencies such as impulsivity and emotion regulation. It follows that clinicians should be alert to how subtle micro relational dynamics may trigger a disproportionate stress response, even in the absence of overt trauma (Perry et al., 1995).

Genes and environment, then, are in constant interaction through epigenetic and relational pathways. This being so, it is increasingly accepted that a child's relational/socio-cultural environment affects brain development. As Winnicott (1965) observed many years ago: "It is this meeting of inherited tendencies with environmental provision that makes for the child's development" (p. 45).

In light of this emergent consensus, I have attempted to balance my preferred psychosocial model by drawing on findings from multiple perspectives that I find compelling, not least attachment theory, neurobiology, and relational neuroscience. The integration of these diverse perspectives is in the service of deepening an understanding of the complex processes under discussion. Although I advocate an integrated approach, it may be accepted that there is now a substantial body of research legitimising psychosocial perspectives without reverting to parent-blaming. Indeed, understanding the processes of transmission can be liberating rather than blaming.

This chapter, then, advances the concept of cumulative trauma as a relational, developmental, and intergenerational process that is encoded procedurally rather than episodically. It argues that explicit trauma in childhood is frequently embedded within such cumulative relational failures.

Before focusing specifically on cumulative trauma, I think it useful to consider the broader range of traumatic experiences, and the different ways in which trauma may be organised and expressed developmentally.

Forms of Trauma and Cultural Considerations

The word *trauma* derives from the Greek meaning "penetration" and "wounding". Traumatic experience results in feelings of intense fear, helplessness, loss of control, and threat of annihilation. Such affective states overwhelm the adaptations that ordinarily provide people with a sense of self-agency, emotional connection, and coherent meaning (Herman, 1992). Moreover, traumatic affect has a disorganising effect on mental functioning, being a significant factor in the manifestation of various forms of psychopathology (Crastnopol, 2015; de Zulueta, 1993; Music, 2024; Schore, 1994; Tyson & Tyson, 1990; van der Kolk & Fisler, 1995; Wilkinson, 2010).

Indeed, the longitudinal study by the Centers for Disease Control and Prevention (CDC) found that adverse childhood experiences (ACEs) are cumulatively traumatising, alter brain development, affect the body's response to stress, and negatively impact lifelong health. The CDC's Vitalsigns factsheet states "ACEs are linked to chronic health problems, mental illness, and substance misuse in adulthood" (Centers for Disease Control and Prevention, 2019).

Trauma occurs in reaction to a wide range of experiences and can take different forms (Kris, 1956): the unexpected death or loss of a loved person, being violently assaulted, trapped in a fire or caught up in a terrorist incident, being subjected to rape, sexual, or physical abuse, witnessing a violent death, and being exposed to prolonged periods of fear in a war setting. Traumatic experiences such as these have been extensively documented in the literature on post-traumatic stress disorder (PTSD) and complex PTSD, as have the biological and behavioural sequelae and their effects on personality development and neurogenesis (Herman, 1992; van der Kolk, 1994, 2005).

The most pronounced psychobiological reaction to the fear, terror, and helplessness that characterise overt trauma is pathological dissociation – an altered, detached state of consciousness automatically induced by an uncontrolled cascade of stress-related neurochemicals (Cozolino, 2002, 2006). The traumatic experience is thus severed from consciousness, becoming encoded in the systems of implicit memory in the form of sensory fragments with no linking narrative (van der Kolk, 1994; Schacter, 1996; Schore, 2001; Pally, 2005). Therapists may encounter fragmented sensory memories of this kind in child and adult patients, manifested as sudden bodily sensations or affective states without narrative coherence. This signifies the activation of dissociated trauma and requires careful containment. Dissociated trauma, then, is exquisitely vulnerable to somatisation – as van der Kolk (1994) notes, "the body keeps the score" (p. 253). The clinical implications of dissociation and severely compromised regulation are taken up further in Chapter 12.

Trauma may consist of a single event or a repeated pattern of maltreatment, for example, being routinely subjected to physical, sexual or emotional abuse in childhood and adolescence. The latter would come under the rubric of chronic developmental trauma. The way in which trauma is subjectively experienced will, of course, be mediated by various factors: the person's innate constitution, the protective buffer and emotional resilience provided by secure attachment, psychological vulnerability consequent on a disorganised/unresolved attachment state of mind, the person's ethnicity and gender, as well as specific social, cultural and economic factors that may exacerbate existing family stress.

As noted above, it is essential to recognise that the mediating factors that shape traumatic experience operate within broader cultural and systemic contexts. While the fundamental organisation of attachment behaviour – secure, avoidant, ambivalent, and disorganised – appears consistent across cultures (van IJzendoorn & Sagi, 1999), clinicians must exercise cultural sensitivity in assessing what constitutes misattunement within any given cultural context. Crucially, disorganised attachment, which is most closely associated with unresolved trauma and frightening or frightened caregiving, appears across all cultures studied and remains the pattern most strongly predictive of psychopathology, regardless of cultural context.

An influential attachment-informed account of the intergenerational transmission of Holocaust trauma is provided by Fonagy (1999), who argues that such transmission occurs not primarily through explicit narratives or conscious identification, but through early caregiving relationships shaped by unintegrated traumatic states of mind. Drawing on clinical material, Fonagy suggests that caregivers who are themselves survivors of extreme trauma may struggle to mentalise their own experiences and affects, resulting in frightened or frightening patterns of relating that undermine the infant's capacity for affect regulation and coherent self-organisation.

In this model, traumatic experience is transmitted implicitly, through disruptions in attachment and mentalisation, rather than through direct exposure to traumatic events. Fonagy's formulation is consistent with contemporary understandings of cumulative trauma as procedurally encoded and relationally mediated, and offers a clinically grounded account of how historical and collective trauma may come to shape the psychic organisation of subsequent generations.

Clinicians, then, need to hold a dual awareness: recognising the universal processes by which cumulative trauma develops and is transmitted, while simultaneously understanding how systemic oppression creates neurobiological vulnerability to trauma. As discussed above, chronic exposure to systemic marginalisation functions as an environmental stressor that alters stress-response systems, attachment neurobiology, and regulatory capacities through epigenetic pathways.

Parents facing chronic social and economic marginalisation, navigating hostile environments, or coping with the intergenerational effects of historical trauma are responding to, and being neurobiologically shaped by, systemic failures that threaten the family's wellbeing. The theoretical frameworks presented in this chapter operate across cultural boundaries, but their clinical application requires culturally informed judgment that neither pathologises difference nor attributes genuine suffering to cultural factors when systemic injustice and its biological consequences are at play.

The Coexistence of Explicit Trauma and Cumulative Trauma

Whether a single event or a repeated pattern, the various forms of trauma outlined in this section are generally seen as being overt and explicit, and therefore as occurring in the verbal, conscious domain. That said, from my clinical experience in both the criminal justice system and private practice, it is important to note that explicit and cumulative forms of trauma are not mutually exclusive and may frequently coexist. In cases of chronic intrafamilial maltreatment, such as repeated sexual abuse, physical violence, or coercive control, overt traumatic events typically occur within a relational context already characterised by profound failures of attunement, empathy, and mentalisation.

Such abuse requires the caregiver to override or remain unresponsive to the child's signals of distress, relating to the child as an object rather than as a subject with an inner life (Ferenczi, 1933). From a contemporary developmental perspective, explicit trauma in childhood is often embedded within, and made possible by, an underlying matrix of cumulative trauma. The ways in which such early objectifying dynamics may later become sexualised and enacted within the therapeutic relationship are explored in Chapter 11.

By contrast, in the absence of overt abuse, cumulative trauma may arise *solely* through chronic misattunement, emotional unavailability, and failures of repair within otherwise "good enough" caregiving environments. The clinical presentation of these different configurations varies accordingly, with explicit trauma often associated with dissociation and fragmentation, and cumulative trauma more commonly shaping rigid or constricted patterns of affect regulation, attachment states, and intimate relationships.

Within this broader range of traumatic experience, cumulative trauma warrants particular attention as a relational and developmental process that accrues gradually, often without any single event that can be readily named or remembered. The following sections explore in greater detail how repeated experiences of misattunement and relational disruption shape development over time.

Cumulative Trauma, Implicit Memory, and the Child's Experience of Non-influence

As noted in the introduction, cumulative trauma refers to the developmental impact of repeated, unaddressed disruptions in early relational experience. These may occur in the absence of discrete traumatic events. Rather than being organised around conscious, episodic memory, cumulative trauma is encoded procedurally within implicit memory, shaping expectations of self and others and patterns of relating, as well as the capacity for affect regulation and mentalisation. Cumulative trauma is transmitted intergenerationally, not through explicit narratives of trauma, but through embodied, non-verbal, and largely implicit patterns of interaction that are enacted within attachment relationships. In this sense, cumulative trauma is not an accumulation of events, but the progressive structuring of relational experience over time. These cumulative patterns not only shape how the child adapts moment by moment, they also influence the broader relational expectations that quietly consolidate over time.

The child's repeated experience of being unable to influence their caregiver is a subtle but deeply shaping form of cumulative trauma. When a caregiver remains psychologically unmoved – unresponsive to the child's signals, affects, or bids for connection – the child learns that their internal states have little impact on the relational world. Over time, this chronic non-contingency becomes an organising experience: distress does not bring comfort, joy does not evoke pride and shared delight, and protest does not alter anything. What is internalised is not simply insecurity but a felt sense of relational inefficacy, a quiet conviction that one cannot influence another mind or meaningfully affect what happens (Lyons-Ruth et al., 2005; Beebe et al., 2000).

This absence of relational influence becomes embodied, shaping both neurobiological calibration and the child's emerging sense of self. Stress-response systems adapt to a world in which signalling is futile. This fosters patterns of emotional minimisation, hyper-adaptation, or resignation. Clinically, these show up as diminished agency, difficulty in asserting needs, or a pervasive sense of not being kept in mind. In therapy, there is often a transference enactment informed by the implicit belief that the therapist will remain unmoved by the patient's plight. However, moments in which the therapist is genuinely affected and emotionally touched by the patient can be powerfully transformative, offering a profoundly new relational experience. Attending to these dynamics allows us to recognise how early relational futility becomes woven into later clinical presentations, often in ways that are subtle, tenacious, and easily overlooked.

In contrast to overt, explicit trauma, interest in this more subtle, nuanced form of trauma, which, by developmental default, may be preverbal, emerged during the past 50 years. The focus here is on infant development and early caregiver-infant interaction patterns. To the untrained eye, the form of cumulative trauma that came to be studied is largely silent and invisible, being unwittingly transmitted from parent to infant, predominantly in the implicit-procedural domain of being-and-relating (Beebe & Lachmann, 1992; Beebe et al., 2000; Renn, 2012; Schacter, 1987; Stern et al., 1998). While pathological dissociation is a pronounced characteristic of acute trauma, cumulative trauma, being more typically encoded procedurally, does not have the fragmentation seen in dissociative presentations. However, where the misattunement is chronic, this may produce dissociative defences, especially in highly sensitive children.

In clinical work, these implicit relational patterns may manifest as repetitive play themes, characteristic ways of managing separation and reunion, difficulty with transitions, or rigid patterns of response to the therapist's affective bids. The child cannot typically articulate these patterns – they are enacted rather than narrated.

Although implicit memory is acquired and employed in a largely nonconscious way, it may, nonetheless, vitally influence our thoughts, feelings and behaviours. Such memories arise in early development as a natural consequence of everyday repetitive and habitual experiences as perceiving, relating and acting. Implicit memories structure our inner world, as variously conceptualised as internal working models, relational configurations, scripts, schemas, and object relations. Nonconscious, implicit modes of interaction are enacted, for good or for ill, in our most intense intimate relationships. In this sense, implicit memory operates as a set of embodied predictions and relational scripts. Cumulative trauma compromises implicit memory systems and disrupts the development of flexible autonomic regulation. This leaves the child oscillating between states of hyper-arousal and hypo-arousal as adaptive but costly survival strategies.

In both child and adult psychotherapy, repetitive relational enactments can be understood as implicit memory in action. Recognising these patterns helps clinicians to make links and intervene at the level of lived relational experience, rather than explicit recollection. An example of this may be seen in my work with Patricia in chapter 9. This vignette emphasises again that cumulative trauma needs to be understood not as an accumulation of *events*, but as the progressive shaping of implicit expectations about the self in relationship with others. I draw attention to this distinction in Chapter 6, where I compare Brewin et al.'s (1996) "dual processing theory" with the relational-neurodevelopmental framework I am proposing.

Contemporary Psychoanalytic Developments

Psychoanalytic theory offers an early and nuanced framework for understanding cumulative trauma as a disturbance in the continuity of emotional experience. Commenting on the genesis of the infant mental health movement, Arietta Slade (2023) suggests that this may be said to lie in Fraiberg et al.'s (1975) paradigm-shifting paper, "Ghosts in the Nursery". This is a classic psychodynamic account of how unresolved trauma in parents reemerges in the caregiving environment. Masud Khan's (1963) theory of "cumulative trauma" is also influential in this context. Khan's (1963) concept of cumulative trauma is informed by the ideas that Freud (1920) set out in *Beyond the Pleasure Principle*, namely that a protective shield functions to protect the immature ego from excitations from the external world.

Whereas Freud (1920) construed this capacity as a function of the ego, Khan (1963), in a more relational way, emphasised the infant's dependence on the mother (caregiver), and her role as a protective shield and auxiliary ego throughout development. Khan would have been aware of Freud's (1926) concept of "primal repression" – an early form of repression manifested in intense archaic experiences that break through the protective shield.

Khan was closely allied to Winnicott, and also to Anna Freud, who championed his thinking. His elaboration of Freud's protective shield theory is also apparent in Winnicott's (1958) view that the mother's role is to present the outside world to the infant in a way that preserves the illusion of omnipotence, thereby protecting the child from precipitate disillusionment and traumatic impingements. In his final paper, Winnicott (1974) drew a distinction between the Freudian repressed unconscious, on the one hand, and unremembered unconscious phenomena from early childhood, on the other hand – the ghosts in the nursery?

Lacan (1993) subsequently theorised primal repression as a form of memory that remains inaccessible to the person. In this sense, primal repression, and the theory that repetitive actions are a form of unconscious memory (Freud, 1914, 1926), may be seen as having certain phenomenal features in common with the performative, emotional, and enactive aspects of implicit memory (Reis, 2009). Similarly, Fonagy and Target (1997) argue that screen memories, as theorised by Freud (1914), may be conceptualised as a manifestation of the implicit-procedural memory system "which can achieve no other phenomenal representation" (p. 215).

Fraiberg, Adelson, and Shapiro's (1975) seminal paper challenged the oft unquestioned view that parents are naturally and universally benign and protective of their infants. Every nursery, they argue, has its ghosts, that is, uninvited visitors from the parents' unremembered past. In favourable circumstances, the bond of love between parent and infant is protective of their relationship and facilitates the banishment of the unbidden, malevolent spirits. But how to explain the fact that other, less fortunate families become possessed by their ancestral ghosts, with the consequence that their family tragedy is endlessly rehearsed from a well-worn script?

A further significant contribution that enriches our understanding of how parental psychobiological states become internalised comes from André Green's (1983) formulation of the "dead mother complex". This provides a powerful account of how a caregiver's depression or emotional withdrawal impacts the child. Green observed that when a previously attuned mother becomes psychically absent – often following her own loss or trauma – the infant experiences a sudden collapse of the mother's emotional availability.

Although the mother remains physically present, her affective presence is felt to have "died". Crucially, Green argued that the infant does not simply register this withdrawal, but internalises the mother's deadened state as a "dead object" within the psyche. While this may be said to be a specific form of cumulative trauma, in that it is characterised by a sudden affective withdrawal, the process of internalisation would be gradual. In this sense, the child's experience may be said to consist of a combination of overt trauma and cumulative trauma, as discussed above.

Green argues that the internalisation of the depressed mother results in a core of psychic emptiness, inhibition of spontaneity, and a defensive split between a "living" and a "dead" part of the self. These dynamics often re-emerge in adulthood as difficulties sustaining intimacy, sudden emotional withdrawal, or a pervasive sense of inner deadness. Clinically, the "dead mother" may appear in the transference as a collapse of affect, a sense of futility, or a fear that the therapist will die or become emotionally unavailable. Green's formulation also resonates with earlier psychoanalytic accounts of fundamental relational disturbance, most notably Balint's concept of the "basic fault", which also describes a pre-symbolic disruption in the fabric of the child's early experience (Balint, 1968).

Green's model thus complements both Khan's and Fraiberg's formulations by illustrating how a parent's depression or emotional withdrawal becomes a form of cumulative trauma, transmitted implicitly and enacted procedurally within the attachment relationship. His work anticipates contemporary developmental accounts by locating trauma not solely in discrete events but in the ongoing relational processes through which the infant's sense of aliveness, desire, and meaning is shaped.

These psychoanalytic formulations, then, anticipate later developmental and attachment-informed accounts by locating trauma in the disruptions of relational processes rather than in isolated events. Thus, from a contemporary perspective, Fraiberg's pertinent question as to why some families remain haunted by their ancestral ghosts may be reframed as follows: What relational processes are involved in the transmission of cumulative trauma from one generation to the next?

Attachment and Intergenerational Transmission

Attachment theory would seem to be the most productive starting point in exploring this question, since a central concern of attachment research is understanding the intergenerational transmission of attachment patterns and states of mind. These findings provide empirical support for psychoanalytic accounts of cumulative trauma, illuminating the micro-processes through which relational patterns are established.

The two main methods used in attachment research are the Strange Situation Procedure (Ainsworth et al., 1978) and the Adult Attachment Interview (George, Kaplan & Main, 1985; Main & Goldwyn, 1995; Main, Kaplan & Cassidy, 1985). These methodologies are designed to induce a degree of stress, thereby activating the attachment system and concomitant representational models. In effect, this research taps into implicit-procedural memory, the dynamics of which are manifested in infant attachment behaviour and adult discourse style (Crittenden, 1990; Fonagy, 1998, 1999; Goldwyn & Hugh-Jones, 2011; Slade, 2004).

Research utilising the strange situation procedure (SSP) found that infants display one of four discrete patterns of attachment behaviour when briefly separated from and reunited with their mothers in the presence of a stranger. These patterns have been classified as secure, avoidant, ambivalent-resistant and disorganised/disoriented. Attachment patterns, and concomitant behavioural strategies, can be predicted to a high level of accuracy from the quality of interaction observed between the primary caregiver and infant during the first year of life (Main, Kaplan & Cassidy, 1985).

Indeed, findings demonstrate that a parent's Adult Attachment Interview (AAI) classification (secure-autonomous, dismissing, preoccupied, or unresolved) predicts child behaviour in the SSP. This, in turn, indicates that attachment is transmitted intergenerationally, being internalised and represented in the form of self-other internal working models (IWMs). These mental models are thought to mediate the infant's experience of actual relationships and guide feelings, behaviour, attention, memory, and cognition largely out of conscious awareness.

In attachment theory the main purpose of defence is the regulation of affect. The primary mechanism for achieving this is "distance regulation" – achieving a balance between proximity seeking and exploration (Sroufe & Waters, 1977). This dilemma is apparent in the different behavioural strategies that insecure infants display in the SSP. Holmes (1993) suggests that both the avoidant and ambivalent strategies employed by infants can be formulated as attachment dilemmas deriving from the need to get close to the attachment figure and the expected dangers of doing so, in terms of rejection, abandonment, inconsistency, or intrusion.

Adult Attachment

The Adult Attachment Interview is a semi-structured interview developed by George, Kaplan, and Main (1985). It provides researchers with a standardised method to assess current adult mental representations of their own childhood attachment experiences, the influence of these experiences as perceived by the interviewee, and the relationship the interviewee has with their parents in the here and now. The participant is also asked about loss of loved ones and other traumatic experiences. The interviewee is faced with the dual task of producing and reflecting upon memories related to attachment, while simultaneously maintaining a coherent discourse with the interviewer.

High levels of coherence indicates that the interviewee has a "singular" rather than a "multiple" representational model of attachment. A single, internally consistent IWM facilitates the integration of attachment-related information and enables the secure individual to explore a wide range of positive and negative thoughts and feelings (Hesse, 1999; Main, 1991). AAI classifications, then, reveal differences in discourse style, in access to attachment memories, and in ability to coherently discuss and reflect on past attachment experience. For clinicians, applying the empirical findings relating to discrete discourse styles can help identify unresolved trauma, as betrayed by narrative incoherence. This, in turn, can guide therapeutic focus towards fostering mentalisation and coherence, thereby enhancing the parent's capacity to reflect on and attune to the child's states.

Combining AAI and SSP Research Methodologies

A long-term study carried out by Main and her colleagues (Main et al., 1985) combined the Adult Attachment Interview and Strange Situation Procedure methodologies. In a follow up study, Main (1991) demonstrated that the child's discrete pattern of attachment organisation has, as its precursor, a characteristic pattern of caregiver-infant interaction and its own behavioural sequelae. Thus, as predicted five years previously, there was a significant match between the mother's AAI classification and her child's SSP classification. In the main, secure-autonomous parents had infants who were securely attached, those with a dismissing state of mind had avoidant infants, while preoccupied parents had ambivalent-resistant infants. There was a strong correlation between caregivers whose discourse transcript was classified as unresolved in respect of abuse and trauma and disorganised/disoriented infants. This robust association pertained even when the AAI was conducted prenatally and the SSP a year after the infant's birth.

Findings indicate that once attachment patterns and states of mind are established, they tend to become actively self-perpetuating. As a consequence, malignant events relevant to attachment may cause difficulty in integrating information. A parent's sensitive responsiveness has consistently been found to be the best predictor of security of attachment at one year of age. Sensitive responsiveness is defined as the capacity of caregivers to correctly appraise the child's attachment signals and respond to them promptly and adequately. By contrast, parental rejection is predictive of infant avoidance, and a parent's inconsistent response predicts ambivalent-resistant infant behaviour. The great majority of parentally maltreated children fit the disorganised/disoriented category (Main & Hesse, 1990; Main, Kaplan & Cassidy, 1985; Main, 1991). What these various findings demonstrate is that cumulative trauma often begins with subtle patterns of misattunement and misrecognition long before trauma is identifiable.

In terms of the mechanisms involved in this process, Main, Kaplan, and Cassidy (1985) suggest that when an established attachment behavioural system receives potentially disruptive signals it counters these by actively deploying perceptual and behavioural control mechanisms. They conclude, albeit tentatively, that internal working models deriving from insecure attachment are resistant to modification and updating because error-correcting information is being defensively and selectively excluded from consciousness.

Significantly, the authors suggest that the difficulty in processing attachment-related information may affect maternal sensitivity, as the need to exclude, restrict or reorganise such information may result in an inability on the part of the mother to perceive and accurately interpret the infant's attachment needs and behaviour. Furthermore, they propose that, because of issues stemming from her own attachment history, the mother may experience an active need to alter or inhibit the signals being expressed by the infant (Main, Kaplan & Cassidy, 1985).

Disruption in Parent–Child Affective Communication

Of relevance here is the finding that it is often not the traumatic event in and of itself that is salient, but rather the characteristic attachment system within which the child experiences the trauma, as alluded to above (Lyons-Ruth & Block, 1996; Lyons-Ruth, Bronfman & Atwood, 1999; Lyons-Ruth et al. 2005; Lyons-Ruth & Jacobvitz, 2008; Renn, 2003, 2012; Rutter, 1997; Settlage et al. 1990). Building on the research by Main et al. (1985), Lyons-Ruth and Block (1996) and Lyons-Ruth et al. (2005) found that women who had been exposed to childhood violence were at elevated risk of emotionally withdrawn caregiving on becoming mothers, and for establishing disorganised attachment with their infants.

Consistent with the concept of cumulative trauma, the authors found that subtle aspects of the relationship seemed to be involved, rather than gross abuse, neglect, or abandonment. This was manifested as profound disruption in patterns of mother-infant verbal and nonverbal affective communication, with repeated infant communication of distress, anger, or contact-seeking being entirely overridden by repetitive non-responsive behaviours by the mothers. Significantly, there was little or no attempt by the mothers to repair the derailed interaction.

Similar dynamics may be apparent in a patient's narrative and style of relating in clinical work with both individuals and couples. For example, bids by the patient's partner for connection are repeatedly met with withdrawal or misattunement. Therapy can help to reveal such maladaptive, procedural forms of relating, and encourage the patient to engage in new, more emotionally connected ways. This can feel daunting and even emotionally dangerous to the patient, but is necessary for the eventual establishment of new, more life-enhancing ways of relating.

Lyons-Ruth and Block (1996) conclude that mothers who had been traumatised in childhood by their attachment figures may use unresponsive withdrawal and unresponsive hostile-intrusiveness in the service of minimising their own responsive emotional contact with their infant. Such behaviour is employed as a means of self-protection to avoid the activation of their own unintegrated traumatic memories.

Indirect displays of fear by the mother evoke fear in the infant whose felt security is directly tied to the communicative adequacy of the maternal relationship. In essence, the attachment behavioural system becomes non-functional, with little or no protective function at the level of infant experience. From this perspective, cumulative trauma emerges through repeated failures of attunement and repair that become encoded in the child's implicit relational world.

Neurobiological Foundations of Cumulative Trauma

Contemporary neurobiological and epigenetic research offers further insight into how early relational experience becomes biologically embedded. The findings from attachment research, as set out in the previous section, reflect Schore's (2011) contention that implicitly encoded preverbal communication is transmitted intergenerationally by means of the psychobiological exchanges embedded in the co-created attachment bond. Moreover, he avers that trauma deriving from dysregulated attachment experiences, as described by Lyons-Ruth and Block (1996), becomes indelibly imprinted in the right brain and is associated with the child's use of dissociation. He cites findings showing that an impaired ability to regulate the intensity of affect is the most enduring consequence of cumulative trauma (Schore, 1994, 2011). Somewhat contentiously, he argues that all early psychopathology constitutes disorders of attachment and is manifested as failures of interactive regulation of preverbal affect (Schore, 1994).

Although rather overstated, both Schore's theory of affect regulation and Porges's (2011) polyvagal theory highlight the way in which infants literally *borrow* the caregiver's nervous system for regulation – that a system of co-regulation is in play throughout early development. This account is consistent with the framework of interpersonal neurobiology, which emphasises that the development of self-regulation emerges through early experiences of co-regulation within attachment relationships (Siegel, 2001, 2012). The transmission of inconsistent, fearful or disorganised parental states leaves the child's nervous system primed for either hyper-arousal or hypo-arousal states. Such states are manifested in later development in the form of attention problems, impulsivity or anxiety, often accompanied by a range of co-morbid symptoms, such as eating disorders, drug/alcohol misuse, and self-injury behaviour.

The Mirror Neuron System

Continuing with a neurobiological perspective, the evocation of fear in the infant via witnessing indirect fear by the mother, as found by Lyons-Ruth, may be seen to reflect the functioning of the mirror neuron system. The mirror neuron circuitry is said to be present at birth and is thought to be the neurobiological substrate for our innate capacity to read and empathically share emotions, intentions, and sensations with others (Rizzolatti, Fogassi & Gallese, 2006). It is thought that the mirror neuron system is activated when we observe the other's actions, intentions, and emotions, taking the form of what Gallese (2009) terms "embodied simulation". In essence, the assertion is that the same neurons fire in the brain of the person observing the actions or emotional display of another as if they were performing the observed action or experiencing the same feelings (Cozolino, 2002).

While these findings are preliminary, and the precise mechanisms remain contentious and under investigation, the suggestion is that the mirror neuron system permits us to participate in the other's actions without having to imitate them (Boston Change Process Study Group, 2008). Such research may help to elucidate the complex processes by which preverbal and nonverbal emotional communication occurs (Cozolino, 2002; Divino & Moore, 2010). In this context, Shai and Belsky (2011) focus on parent–child *embodied* interaction. Introducing the concept of "parental embodied mentalization", they argue that "psychological and neuroscientific work clearly shows that kinaesthetic patterns consistently convey distinct mental states" (p. 175).

Clinicians may observe these transmission processes in the visceral quality of parent–child interactions: the mother who stiffens when her child approaches for comfort, the father whose voice becomes a dull, flat monotone when discussing feelings, the parent who consistently looks away during moments of emotional intensity. Such micro-behaviours, operating outside conscious awareness, carry profound relational meaning.

Such findings reflect a distancing from Descartes's dualism theory, that is a distinction between an immaterial mind and a physical body. Tronick (2007) reframes Descartes's well-known aphorism "I think, therefore I am" as "I interact, therefore I am", as informed by his "still face" studies of infant-parent mutual exchanges. Tronick's relational rephrasing emphasises an existentialist, phenomenological, and social constructivist philosophical position, as opposed to the epistemological certainty that Descartes brings to the salience of solitary thought.

In terms of intergenerational transmission via repetitive patterns of misattuned parent–child interactions, the mirror neuron system may facilitate infants *mapping* parents' affective states directly into their own bodies through non-verbal channels such as tone of voice, facial expression, and body tension. This process reflects the assertion made by various authors in the field of child development that the mind is first embodied, then embedded, then encoded. Repeated cycles of attuned mirroring acts to scaffold the child's own capacity for self-awareness and emotion regulation. This is congruent with Gergely and Watson's (1996) social biofeedback theory, as discussed below.

The long-term consequences of such embodied transmission can be seen clinically in individuals whose early environments were marked by fear, misattunement, or frightening caregiving. In Michael's case, for example, repeated exposure to unresponsive and dysregulated caregivers, combined with traumatic loss and sexual abuse, resulted in the implicit encoding of fear and abandonment. These early, embodied experiences were later reactivated in adulthood under conditions of relational threat, overwhelming his capacity for regulation and mentalisation.

Michael's formative experiences consisted of cumulative relational trauma and dramatic trauma in the form of loss, abandonment, and sexual abuse. In the absence of help to process these experiences, he developed a disorganised attachment pattern and profound difficulty regulating emotional states associated with rejection and abandonment. In adulthood, these dissociated childhood experiences were reactivated under conditions of separation and loss, overwhelming his capacity to mentalise and regulate affect.

Observations from neonatal medicine further underscore the centrality of embodied co-regulation in early development. Skin-to-skin contact between premature infants and their caregivers has been shown to stabilise heart rate and physiological functioning, illustrating how regulation is not an intrinsic capacity of the infant alone, but emerges within an attuned relational context. Such findings highlight the fundamentally embodied and relational nature of early regulation, and provide a physiological analogue to the processes of affective attunement and repair described throughout this chapter.

These findings underscore how cumulative trauma operates at the intersection of relational experience and biological regulation, without implying biological determinism. It follows that the therapist's embodied presence – tone, gaze, posture – can serve as a corrective mirroring experience, supporting affect regulation and mentalisation in patients whose early experiences were dysregulated. More generally, and in addition to the therapeutic relationship itself, enabling the patient to become "earned secure" (Main,

Kaplan & Cassidy, 1985), and enhancing affect regulation and mentalisation, facilitates the transformation of the procedural relational dynamics that characterise cumulative trauma.

The Transmission of Relational Experience and Neural Plasticity

We see, then, that when parents themselves are depressed, dysregulated or behave in frightening ways, the child internalises that psychobiological dysregulation, which shapes their own developing nervous system. Mirror neuron research dovetails with the findings of attachment and epigenetics, helping to reveal how relational experiences are transmitted across generations. These findings also emphasise that biology and psychosocial processes are inextricably entangled – that there is a two-way connection between mind and body (Bullmore, 2018, 2024).

Mirroring processes display neural plasticity and the infant's dependence on the mirroring subject. Although neuroplasticity occurs across the lifecycle, the developing brain is particularly plastic. While this imparts vulnerability to the child, it also means that transformative repair and healing can occur (Cozolino, 2002, 2006). In a similar way to neural plasticity, recent findings indicate epigenetic plasticity for DNA methylation. While previously regarded as a stable inscription, emerging evidence suggests that attuned relational experience – including psychotherapy – may be accompanied by shifts in methylation within stress-regulatory pathways. Although this research remains at an early stage, it indicates that the relational field may participate in epigenetic recalibration (Perroud et al., 2013).

Preliminary research suggests that the capacity for neural mirroring is the neuro-physiological substrate for empathy, as well as facilitating our ability to meaningfully appraise the actions, intentions, and emotions of others. Given this, the mirror neuron system would seem to be linked to the capacity for mentalisation, as discussed below. Indeed, as Jurist and Meehan (2009) point out, mentalisation theory is grounded in ideas from neuroscience and cognitive psychology, a view endorsed by Shai and Belsky (2011).

Mentalisation, Epistemic Trust, Parental Reflective Functioning, and the Transmission Gap

While there is robust evidence supporting the association between adult and child attachment, as well as for the role of parental sensitive responsiveness in influencing child attachment security, parental sensitivity does not fully explain the relation between adult and child attachment (van IJzendoorn, 1995; van IJzendoorn & Bakermans-Kranenburg, 2019). How, then, is this gap in the transmission of attachment to be explained? Parental mentalisation of the child's thoughts and feelings, van IJzendoorn and Bakermans-Kranenburg (2019) suggest, is a plausible starting point, and one that might help to narrow this gap. Moreover, mentalisation provides an additional lens through which the developmental consequences of cumulative trauma may be understood.

Mentalisation is the capacity to interpret the actions and behaviours of oneself and others as meaningful on the basis of intentional mental states, such as personal needs, desires, feelings, beliefs, and purposes (Bateman & Fonagy, 2004). It involves holding multiple perspectives in mind and regulating affect during interpersonal stress. The person's attachment history impacts the ability to mentalise. Securely attached children tend to have high mentalising caregivers, and thus develop robust capacities to represent their own and others' states of mind. Insecure and disorganised attachment consequent on exposure to cumulative trauma with low mentalising caregivers compromises mentalising capacities (Fonagy, 2008; Fonagy et al., 2002). Fonagy (2008) stressed the vicious cycle created by cumulative trauma in hyper-activating the attachment system and closing down mentalisation. Thus, although mentalisation is regarded as a multifaceted and variable process, it is generally agreed that the capacity to mentalise crucially depends on the infant's earliest emotional exchanges with the primary caregiver (Fonagy et al., 2002).

Closely related to mentalisation is the concept of epistemic trust (Fonagy & Allison, 2014; Fonagy et al., 2015). This refers to the capacity to regard knowledge communicated by others as trustworthy, generalisable, and relevant to oneself. Epistemic trust develops when caregivers not only attune to the child's internal states, but also reliably demonstrate themselves as trustworthy sources of information, both about the child's inner world and the external environment. This dual function – affective attunement and reliable communication – helps to establish the child's openness to social learning more broadly.

Cumulative trauma impairs the development of epistemic trust, resulting in a state of hypervigilant suspicion of others. Thus, even in benevolent relationships the child may be unable to accept or integrate new knowledge offered in therapeutic or social contexts. Fonagy and colleagues (Fonagy et al., 2017) term this state "epistemic petrification" – a defensive closure to new information. While this protects against further relational disappointment, it simultaneously forecloses opportunities for growth and change. This partly explain why some patients struggle to benefit from therapy, despite the therapist's genuine attunement and care, and why restoring epistemic trust becomes a central therapeutic task, alongside enhancing mentalisation itself.

Reflective Functioning, the Transmission Gap, and Relationship Specific Attachment

The terms *mentalisation* and *reflective functioning* are often used interchangeably. Reflective functioning refers to a scale devised by Fonagy and his colleagues to operationalise mentalisation for research purposes (Fonagy, et al., 1998). Reflective functioning refers to the capacity to perceive mental states in oneself and others. Slade's research with parents and children in psychotherapy draws a distinction between parental reflective functioning and parental attachment organisation. The former refers to the caregiver's capacity to reflect on the current mental state of the child and on her own mental states as these pertain to her relationship with her child. The latter refers to her capacity to reflect on her childhood relationships with her own parents, as classified by the AAI (Slade, 2005; Slade et al., 2005; Grienenberger, Kelly & Slade, 2005; Slade, 2008).

Slade argues that parental reflective functioning is more influential than parental attachment organisation in terms of predicting positive outcomes, such as secure attachment in the child. This may partly explain why some parents with insecure attachment do not transmit insecure states to their children. Impairments in reflective functioning can thus be seen as both an outcome of cumulative trauma and a mechanism through which it is transmitted across generations.

Indeed, it is suggested that reflective functioning, as variously described by Grienenberger, Kelly, and Slade (2005), Fonagy (2008), Fonagy et al. (2002), and Slade (2008), helps to explain the transmission gap first noted by van IJzendoorn (1995). Therapists can actively cultivate reflective functioning in parents, encouraging curiosity about and exploration of their own and their child's mental states as a way of interrupting cycles of cumulative trauma. Such reparative and mentalising processes constitute therapeutic action in both child and adult psychotherapy.

Although attachment security in the first year of life is predicted primarily by the security of the mother's attachment organisation and level of reflective functioning, Steele and Steele's longitudinal study at University College London found that the father's level of reflective functioning was significantly related to a number of interpersonal and personality factors in the developing child. Steele and Steele (2008) conclude that attachment is "relationship specific", with representational models of mother and father developing separately, rather than as one overarching model of attachment. This accords with Main, Kaplan and Cassidy's (1985) earlier finding showing that a child may be disorganised with one parent but not with the other.

Developmental Processes: Linking Early Relational Disruptions to Cumulative Trauma

The processes involved in the intergenerational transmission of discrete patterns of interactive regulation have been illuminated by infant research. This has demonstrated that subtle, fine-grain interactive micro-behaviours are related to intersubjectivity, attachment, and the transmission of emotion from one generation to the next. Such micro-behaviours operate at the level of implicit relational knowing (Boston Change Process Study Group, 2008;

Stern et al., 1998) and include the co-ordination of gaze direction, vocal inflections, body posture, and facial expressions. These findings illustrate that the intergenerational transmission of cumulative trauma occurs largely outside conscious awareness, via implicit relational patterns rather than explicit communication.

The infant perceives and remembers the caregiver's repetitive subtle behaviours in the form of pre-symbolic interactional expectancies, as illustrated in Chapter 3. Thus, the cumulative impact of repeated interactions that are consistently matched or mismatched creates a structuring effect on the infant, for good or for ill, who then generalises these pre-symbolic representations of interactional expectancies to other interpersonal contexts (Stern, 1985; Beebe, et al., 1985; Beebe & Lachmann, 1992; Beebe, Jaffe & Lachmann, 1992; Knox, 1999, 2001; Marrone, 2014; Peck, 2003; Renn, 2008, 2012; Teicholz, 2009).

Micro-interactions and the Development of Mental Models

As previously emphasised, trauma is not only a matter of discrete, overt events, but a consequence of repeated micro-interactions – failures of attunement, inconsistent mirroring, and chronic misrecognition – that shape implicit models of self and others that are carried into later life. In other words, cumulative trauma is passed on not as remembered experience, but as lived expectation within ongoing relationships.

The caregiver's timing, tracking, and coordination of interactive regulation occurs in the implicit/enactive domain. Secure attachment and optimal self-regulation of affect is facilitated when the coordination is neither too low (avoidant) nor too high (enmeshed). Mid-range coordination that is contingent and predictable, yet flexible and variable, is optimal as it promotes a sense of felt security and thus the capacity to experience new information and relationship transformations (Beebe et al., 2000).

In child psychotherapy, the therapist's attuned, contingent relationship with the child may facilitate a transformation from an overly rigid way of thinking, feeling and engaging in the world to a more playful, flexible style. This, in turn, helps the child to regulate affective states, such as separation anxiety, such that the child can sleep away from home and their parents. It is by encouraging the patient, child or adult, to repeatedly take risks which challenge implicitly encoded archaic ways of functioning that new procedural models are developed, together with an enhanced sense of felt security, and capacity for affect regulation.

Rupture and Repair, and the Social Biofeedback Model

Beebe, Jaffe, and Lachmann (1992) conceptualise misattunement as the loss of mutual influence or contingent responsivity. Research indicates that the infant may come to associate lack of contingency with negative affect and escalating arousal. This, in turn, may interfere with the infant's optimal regulation of their arousal. The authors suggest that prolonged and severe states of withdrawal to accomplish re-regulation of arousal in the face of misattuned caregiving may compromise the infant's attention and information processing capacities. They argue that an infant who typically uses inhibition of responsivity alters their capacity to stay alert and to be fully attentive and responsive to the environment. To preclude this from happening, Beebe and Lachmann (1994) emphasise the need to repair misattunement ruptures in a timely and adequate way.

Similarly, Tronick et al., (1978), informed by their "still face" research, as noted above, conclude that the micro-repair of the breakdown of attunement or misaligned interaction is at the heart of the establishment of a viable human relationship. The establishment of this form of relational sensibility can help patients to develop new empathic connections with their children and partners, together with a new curiosity about their emotional lives.

The findings of infant research align with Gergely and Watson's (1996) social biofeedback theory of parental affect-mirroring from a psychology perspective. Their theory provides a framework for understanding how affective processes mediate the intergenerational transmission of cumulative trauma. They propose that the caregiver's *marked* and *contingent* mirroring of the infant's emotional expressions functions as a form of social biofeedback. This enables the infant to perceive and gradually internalise coherent representations of affective experience. Through such repetitive, attuned interactions, the infant learns to recognise, name, and regulate emotions, thereby establishing the foundations of a stable sense of self and affective agency.

However, when this mirroring process is disrupted – whether through chronic misattunement, parental emotional unavailability, or the parent's own history of unresolved trauma – the infant receives inconsistent or unmarked reflections of their inner states. These distortions undermine the development of integrated affect representations and thus compromise emerging capacities for self-regulation. Such unwitting failures of affect-mirroring can give rise to enduring patterns of emotion dysregulation, vulnerability to stress, and a fragile, fragmented sense of self.

Gergely and Watson's (1996) model illuminates the implicit, nuanced processes involved in the gradual development of cumulative trauma, and the way in which such trauma may be transmitted across generations. Significantly, the processes of transmission are not only via behavioural repetition or explicit communication, but also through subtle failures in emotional feedback systems that shape the earliest forms of self-experience.

Convergence of Psychosocial and Biological Models

These respective perspectives, then, show that patterns of interactive regulation emerge moment-by-moment, being mediated by the caregiver's attachment state of mind, level of reflective functioning, and capacity for contingent marking and mirroring (Beebe et al., 2005; Fonagy & Target, 1996, 1998; Fonagy et al., 2002; Fonagy, 2008; Gergely & Watson, 1996; Slade, 2008). Repeated patterns of optimal or sub-optimal interpersonal experience are encoded in the child's implicit-procedural memory and conceptualised as self-other representational models. A salient aspect of these largely non-conscious mental models consists of generalised beliefs, predictions, and expectations about relationships between the self and key attachment figures, not the least of which concerns one's worthiness to receive love and care (Bowlby, 1998, 1988).

This chapter argues that developmental and psychological perspectives have much in common with neurobiological and epigenetic findings, which, in turn, points to a convergence between psychosocial and biological models. The proposition that genetics and the environment are in opposition, with each providing distinct, discrete explanations would seem to be an increasingly false dichotomy. As Bullmore (2018, 2024) has argued, the persistent division between biological and psychosocial models reflects an outdated mind-body dualism rather than contemporary evidence.

Conclusion

Cumulative trauma is best understood as a relational and developmental process that becomes woven into the fabric of implicit memory long before the child can think or speak about experience. It is transmitted not through dramatic events but through repeated experiences of misattunement, affect dysregulation, and failures of repair that gradually shape relational expectations. These patterns are enacted procedurally, carried in the body, and passed across generations through the subtle, implicit ways caregivers respond to their children.

The convergence of psychoanalytic theory, attachment research, neurobiology, and epigenetics demonstrated in this chapter provides a coherent framework for understanding how these processes unfold. Each perspective highlights a different facet of the same phenomenon: the ways in which early relational environments organise regulatory capacities, expectations of others, and the development of the self. Crucially, this integrative model allows us to recognise cumulative trauma without resorting to parent-blaming or biological determinism. It situates development within a matrix of relational, cultural, and systemic forces, acknowledging that caregivers themselves are shaped by histories of trauma, social adversity, and structural inequity.

Clinically, in work with both children and adults, this understanding shifts the focus from uncovering discrete traumatic events to working with the lived, moment-to-moment patterns that emerge, both in the therapeutic relationship and in the patient's everyday life. It is in the revelation of these enactments that ghosts from the past become visible, and where new relational possibilities can be co-created. The task is not simply to interpret but to participate – to offer a different kind of experience in which affect can be held, repaired, and made thinkable, thereby facilitating new ways of engaging with partners and children. The clinical dynamics of enactment that arise from these moment-to-moment patterns are examined in detail in Chapter 10.

If cumulative trauma is transmitted through the quiet repetition of misattuned interactions, its healing similarly occurs through the repeated experience of attunement, recognition, and repair, together with new knowledge of the self. In this sense, psychotherapy becomes a site of new developmental accomplishments, where implicit relational knowledge is gradually reorganised and new procedural expectations take root. The work is slow and often subtle but Fraiberg's malignant ghosts can indeed be transformed into Lieberman's "benevolent angels" (Lieberman et al., 2005).

In this sense, the therapeutic process described here may be understood as part of a long psychoanalytic lineage that has emphasised the transformative potential of new emotional experience within an ongoing relational context – now conceptualised less as a discrete corrective event than as a cumulative, implicitly encoded process grounded in sustained attunement and repair.

Taken together, the ideas developed in this chapter establish cumulative relational trauma as a multi-layered phenomenon shaped by early caregiving, implicit memory, neurobiological adaptation, and the broader cultural and systemic contexts in which families live. Understanding trauma in this way allows clinicians to recognise how early relational patterns are carried forward into later development and enacted within therapeutic encounters. This integrative framework prepares the ground for the subsequent chapters, where the clinical implications of these processes are explored in depth – particularly in relation to enactment, boundary complexity, sexuality, and severe disturbance. Throughout the volume, the same developmental and relational principles recur: that trauma is transmitted implicitly, that it becomes visible in patterns of relating, and that therapeutic change emerges through recognition, regulation, and repair. However, if cumulative trauma is encoded procedurally and outside conscious awareness, this raises fundamental questions about memory, representation, and the mechanisms through which therapeutic change becomes possible, questions that are addressed in Chapter 6.

A Poetic Epilogue

First, given the conceptual density of this chapter, it would seem appropriate to end on a lighter, poetic note. While this has a jaundiced tint, it is nevertheless germane to the thesis of this chapter. Philip Larkin's most quoted poem, "This Be the Verse", opens with the famously blunt line: "They fuck you up, your mum and dad" (Larkin, 1974). As he makes clear, they do not mean to, but they pass on all "the faults they had", even adding some extra "just for you".

In three epigrammatic stanzas, Larkin captures the texture of intergenerational transmission: the ordinary, repetitive relational moments that silently shape the emotional world of the child and echo into the next generation. Larkin's personal solution to the fact that so many nurseries become inhabited by ghosts from parents' unremembered past was a stark and sardonic one, articulated in the final line of the poem: "And don't have any kids yourself."

Fortunately, we now have a far richer understanding of these processes, and with it, pathways for transformation that were unavailable to Larkin and his generation. As our knowledge deepens, so too will our capacity to offer patients relational experiences that reshape and transform what was once felt to be inevitable.

Note

1 Readers unfamiliar with specialised terminology may wish to consult the Glossary at the end of this volume.

References

Ainsworth, M. D. S., Blehar, M. C., Waters, E. & Wall, S. (1978). *Patterns of attachment: A psychological study of the strange situation*. Hillsdale, NJ: Erlbaum.

Balint, M. (1968). *The basic fault: Therapeutic aspects of regression*. London: Tavistock Publications.

Bateman, A. & Fonagy, P. (2004). *Psychotherapy for borderline personality disorder: Mentalization-based treatment*. Oxford: Oxford University Press.

Beebe, B., Jaffe, J., Feldstein, S., Mays, K. & Alson, D. (1985). Interpersonal timing: The application of an adult dialogue model to mother-infant vocal and kinesic interactions. In T. Field and N. Fox (eds), *Social perception in infants* (pp. 217–247). Norwood, NJ: Ablex.

Beebe, B. & Lachmann, F. M. (1992). The contribution of mother-infant mutual influence to the origins of self- and object representations. In N. J. Skolnick & S. C. Warshaw (eds), *Relational perspectives in psychoanalysis* (pp. 83–117). Hillsdale, NJ: Analytic Press.

Beebe, B., Jaffe, J. & Lachmann, F. M. (1992). A dyadic systems view of communication. In N. J. Skolnick & S. C. Warshaw (eds), *Relational perspectives in psychoanalysis* (pp. 61–81). Hillsdale, NJ: Analytic Press.

Beebe, B. & Lachmann, F. M. (1994). Representation and internalization in infancy: Three principles of saliency. *Psychoanalytic Psychology*, 11, 127–165.

Beebe, B., Jaffe, J., Lachmann, F. M., Feldstein, S., Crown, C. & Jasnow, M. (2000). Systems models in development and psychoanalysis: The case of vocal rhythm coordination and attachment. *Infant Mental Health Journal*, 21, 99–122.

Beebe, B., Lachmann, F. M. & Jaffe, J. (2000). Mother-infant interaction structures and pre-symbolic self and object representations. *Psychoanalytic Dialogues*, 7(2), 133–182.

Beebe, B., Knoblauch, S., Rustin, J. & Sorter, D. (2005). *Forms of intersubjectivity in infant research and adult treatment: A systems view*. New York: Other Press.

Boomsma, D. I., Busjahn, A. & Peltonen, C. (2002). Classical twin studies and beyond. *Nature Reviews Genetics*, 3(11), 872–882.

Boston Change Process Study Group. (2008). Forms of relational meaning: Issues in the relations between the implicit and reflective-verbal domains. *Psychoanalytic Dialogues*, 18(2), 125–148.

Bowlby, J. (1998). *Attachment and loss, vol. 2: Separation: Anger and anxiety*. London: Pimlico.

Bowlby, J. (1988). *A secure base: Clinical applications of attachment theory*. London: Routledge.

Brewin, C. R., Dalgleish, T. & Joseph, S. (1996). A dual representation theory of posttraumatic stress disorder. *Psychological Review*, 103(4), 670–686.

Bullmore, E. (2018). *The inflamed mind: A radical new approach to depression*. London: Allen Lane.

Bullmore, E. (2024). *The divided mind: Why good mental health means whole person care*. London: Profile Books.

Centers for Disease Control and Prevention. (2019). *Adverse childhood experiences (ACEs)*. Vitalsigns, November. Atlanta, GA: CDC.

Cozolino, L. J. (2002). *The neuroscience of psychotherapy: Building and rebuilding the human brain*. New York: Norton.

Cozolino, L. J. (2006). *The neuroscience of human relationships: Attachment and the developing social brain*. New York: Norton.

Crastnopol, M. (2015). *A psychoanalytic understanding of cumulative psychic injury*. New York: Routledge.

Crittenden, P. M. (1990). Internal representational models of attachment relationships. *Infant Mental Health Journal*, 11, 259–277.

de Zulueta, F. (1993). *From pain to violence: The traumatic roots of destructiveness*. London: Whurr Publications.

Divino, C. L. and Moore, M. S. (2010). Integrating neurobiological findings into psychodynamic psychotherapy training and practice. *Psychoanalytic Dialogues*, 20, 337–355.

Ferenczi, S. (1933). Confusion of tongues between adults and the child. In M. Balint (ed.), *Final contributions to the problems and methods of psycho-analysis* (pp. 156–167). London: Karnac Books.

Fonagy, P. (1998). Moments of change in psychoanalytic theory: Discussion of a new theory of psychic change. *Infant Mental Health Journal*, 19(3), 346–353.

Fonagy, P. (1999). The transgenerational transmission of Holocaust trauma. *Attachment & Human Development*, 1(1), 92–114.

Fonagy, P. (2008). The mentalization-focused approach to social development. In F. N. Busch (ed.), *Mentalization: Theoretical considerations, research findings, and clinical implications* (pp. 3–56). Hove: Analytic Press.

Fonagy, P. & Allison, E. (2014). The role of mentalizing and epistemic trust in the therapeutic relationship. *Psychotherapy*, 51(3), 372–380.

Fonagy, P., Gergely, G., Jurist, E. L. & Target, M. (2002). *Affect regulation, mentalization, and the development of the self*. New York: Other Press.

Fonagy, P., Luyten, P. & Allison, E. (2015). Epistemic petrification and the restoration of epistemic trust: A new conceptualization of borderline personality disorder and its psychosocial treatment. *Journal of Personality Disorders*, 29(5), 575–609.

Fonagy, P., Luyten, P., Allison, E. & Campbell, C. (2017). What we have changed our minds about: Part 2. Borderline personality disorder, epistemic trust and the developmental significance of social communication. *Borderline Personality Disorder and Emotion Dysregulation*, 4, article 9.

Fonagy, P. & Target, M. (1996). Playing with reality: I. Theory of mind and the normal development of psychic reality. *International Journal of Psychoanalysis*, 77 (2), 217–233.

Fonagy, P. & Target, M. (1997). Perspectives on the recovered memory debate. In J. Sandler & P. Fonagy (eds), *Recovered memories of abuse: True or false?* (pp. 183–216). London: Karnac Books.

Fonagy, P. & Target, M. (1998). An interpersonal view of the infant. In A. Hurry (ed.), *Psychoanalysis and developmental therapy* (pp. 3–31). London: Karnac Books.

Fonagy, P., Target, M., Steele, H. & Steele, M. (1998). *Reflective-functioning manual, version 5.0, for application to adult attachment interviews*. London: University College London.

Fraiberg, S., Edelson, E. & Shapiro, V. (1975). Ghosts in the nursery: A psychoanalytic approach to the problems of impaired infant-mother relationships. *Journal of the American Academy of Child Psychiatry*, 14(3), 387–421.

Freud, S. (1914). Remembering, repeating and working-through. In J. Strachey (ed.), *The standard edition of the complete psychological works of Sigmund Freud*, vol. 12 (pp. 145–156). London: Hogarth Press.

Freud, S. (1920). Beyond the pleasure principle. In J. Strachey (ed.), *The standard edition of the complete psychological works of Sigmund Freud*, vol. 18 (pp. 7–64). London: Hogarth Press.

Freud, S. (1926). Inhibitions, symptoms and anxiety. In J. Strachey (ed.), *The standard edition of the complete psychological works of Sigmund Freud*, vol. 20 (pp. 77–174). London: Hogarth Press.

Gallese, V. (2009). Mirror neurons, embodied simulation, and the neural basis of social identification. *Psychoanalytic Dialogues*, 19, 519–536.

George, C., Kaplan, N. & Main, M. (1985). Adult attachment interview. APA PsycTests. doi:10.1037/t02879-000

Gergely, G. & Watson, J. (1996). The social biofeedback theory of parental affect-mirroring: The development of emotional self-awareness and self-control in infancy. *International Journal of Psychoanalysis*, 77, 1181–1212.

Goldwyn, R. & Hugh-Jones, S. (2011). Using the adult attachment interview to understand reactive attachment disorder: Findings from a 10-case adolescent sample. *Attachment & Human Development*, 13(2), 169–191.

Green, A. (1983). The dead mother. *International Journal of Psychoanalysis*, 64, 289–299.

Grienenberger, J., Kelly, K. & Slade, A. (2005). Maternal reflective functioning, mother-infant affective communication, and infant attachment: Exploring the link between mental states and observed caregiving behaviour in the intergenerational transmission of attachment. *Attachment & Human Development*, 7(3), 299–311.

Herman, J. L. (1992). *Trauma and recovery*. New York: Basic Books.

Hesse, E. (1999). The adult attachment interview: Historical and current perspectives. In J. Cassidy & P. R. Shaver (eds), *Handbook of attachment: Theory, research, and clinical applications* (pp. 395–433). New York: Guilford Press.

Heijmans, B. T., Tobi, E. W., Stein, A. D., Putter, H., Blauw, G. J., Susser, E. S., Slagboom, P. E. & Lumey, L. H. (2008). Persistent epigenetic differences associated with prenatal exposure to famine in humans. *Proceedings of the National Academy of Sciences*, 105(44), 17046–17049.

Holmes, J. (1993). *John Bowlby and attachment theory*. London: Routledge.

Jurist, E. L. & Meehan, K. B. (2009). Attachment, mentalization, and reflective functioning. In J. H. Obegi and E. Berant (eds), *Attachment theory and research in clinical work with adults* (pp. 71–93). New York: Guilford Press.

Khan, M. M. R. (1963). The concept of cumulative trauma. *The Psychoanalytic Study of the Child*, 18(1), 286–306.

Knox, J. (1999). The relevance of attachment theory to a contemporary Jungian view of the internal world. *Journal of Analytical Psychology*, 44(4), 511–530.

Kris, E. (1956). The recovery of childhood memories in psychoanalysis. *The Psychoanalytic Study of the Child*, 11(1), 54–88.

Lacan, J. (1993). *The seminar of Jacques Lacan: Book 3: The psychoses 1955–1956*. (ed. J. A. Miller, trans. J. Forrester). New York: Norton.

Larkin, P. (1974). This be the verse. In P. Larkin, *High windows*. London: Faber & Faber.

Lieberman, A. F., Padron, E., Van Horn, P. & Harris, W. W. (2005). Angels in the nursery: The intergenerational transmission of benevolent parental influences. *Infant Mental Health Journal*, 26(6), 504–520.

Lyons-Ruth, K. & Block, D. (1996). The disturbed caregiving system: Relations among childhood trauma, maternal caregiving, and infant affect and attachment. *Infant Mental Health Journal*, 17(3), 257–275.

Lyons-Ruth, K., Bronfman, E. & Atwood, G. (1999). A relational diathesis model of hostile–helpless states of mind: Expressions in mother-infant interaction. In J. Solomon and C. George (eds), *Attachment disorganization* (pp. 33–70). New York: Guilford Press.

Lyons-Ruth, K., Bruschweiler-Stern, N., Harrison, A. M., Morgan, A. C., Nahum, J. P., Sander, L. W., Stern, D. N. & Tronick, E. Z. (1998). Implicit relational knowing: Its role in development and psychoanalytic treatment. *Infant Mental Health Journal*, 19(3), 282–289.

Lyons-Ruth, K., Yellin, C., Melnick, S. & Atwood, G. (2005). Expanding the concept of unresolved mental states: Hostile/helpless states of mind on the adult attachment interview are associated with atypical maternal behaviour and infant disorganization. *Development and Psychopathology*, 17, 1–23.

Lyons-Ruth, K. & Jacobvitz, D. (2008). Attachment disorganization: Genetic factors, parenting contexts, and developmental transformation from infancy to adulthood. In J. Cassidy & P. R. Shaver (eds), *Handbook of attachment: Theory, research, and clinical applications* (2nd edn, pp. 666–697). New York: Guilford Press.

Main, M. & Goldwyn, S. (1995). Interview-based adult attachment classifications: Related to infant-mother and infant-father attachment. *Developmental Psychology*, 19, 227–239.

Main, M., Kaplan, N. & Cassidy, J. (1985). Security in infancy, childhood, and adulthood: A move to the level of representation. In I. Bretherton & E. Waters (eds), *Growing points in attachment: Theory and research* (pp. 66–104). Monographs of the Society for Research in Child Development. Chicago, IL: University of Chicago Press.

Main, M. & Hesse, E. (1990). Parents' unresolved traumatic experiences are related to infant disorganized attachment status: Is frightening and/or frightened parental behaviour the linking mechanism? In M. Greenberg, D. Cicchetti & E. M.

Cummings (eds), *Attachment in the preschool years: Theory, research and intervention* (pp. 161–182). Chicago, IL: University of Chicago Press.

Main, M. (1991). Metacognitive knowledge, metacognitive monitoring, and singular (coherent) vs multiple (incoherent) models of attachment: Findings and directions for future research. In C. M. Parkes, J. Stevenson-Hinde & P. Marris (eds), *Attachment across the life cycle* (pp. 127–159). Hove: Routledge.

Marrone, M. (2014). *Attachment and interaction: From Bowlby to current clinical theory and practice* (2nd ed.). London: Jessica Kingsley Publishers.

Meaney, M. J. (2010). Epigenetics and the biological definition of gene × environment interactions. *Child Development*, 81(1), 41–79.

Music, G. (2024). Brainy kids skating on thin ice: New thoughts on psyche-soma and how minds over-develop to cope with trauma. *The Psychoanalytic Study of the Child*, 77(1), 41–59.

Pally, R. (2005). A neuroscience perspective on forms of intersubjectivity in infant research and adult treatment. In B. Beebe, S. Knoblauch, J. Rustin and D. Sorter (eds), *Forms of intersubjectivity in infant research and adult treatment: A systems view* (pp. 191–241). New York: Other Press.

Peck, C. J. (2003). Patterns of relating in the analytic field. *Psychoanalytic Inquiry*, 23 (2), 202–223.

Perry, B. D., Pollard, R. A., Blakely, T. L., Baker, W. L. & Vigilante, D. (1995). Childhood trauma, the neurobiology of adaptation, and "use-dependent" development of the brain: How "states" become "traits". *Infant Mental Health Journal*, 16, 271–291.

Polderman, T. J. C., Benjamin, B., de Leeuw, C. A., Sullivan, P. F., van Bochoven, A., Visscher, P. M. & Posthuma, D. (2015). Meta-analysis of the heritability of human traits based on fifty years of twin studies. *Nature Genetics*, 47, 702–709.

Porges, S. W. (2011). *The polyvagal theory: Neurophysiological foundations of emotions, attachment, communication, and self-regulation*. New York: W. W. Norton.

Perroud, N. A., Salzmann, A., Prada, P. B., Nicastro, R., Hoeppli Puathy, M.-E., Furrer, S., Ardu, S., Krejci, I., Karege, F. & Malafosse, A. (2013). Response to psychotherapy in borderline personality disorder is associated with methylation changes of the BDNF gene. *Translational Psychiatry*, 3, e207.

Princess of Wales, HRH & Waldinger, R. (2025). *The power of human connection in a distracted world*. London: Royal Foundation Centre for Early Childhood.

Reis, B. (2009). Performative and enactive features of psychoanalytic witnessing: The transference as the scene of address. *International Journal of Psychoanalysis*, 90, 1359–1372.

Renn, P. (2003). The link between childhood trauma and later violent offending: The application of attachment theory in a probation setting. In F. Pfäfflin & G. Adshead (eds), *A matter of security: The application of attachment theory to forensic psychiatry and psychotherapy* (pp. 109–144). London: Jessica Kingsley Publishers.

Renn, P. (2008). Attachment, affect regulation and trauma: The transmission of patterns across generations. In E. Arnold & B. Hawkes (eds), *Internalising the historical past: Issues for separation and moving on* (pp. 24–33). Newcastle: Cambridge Scholars Publishing.

Renn, P. (2012). *The silent past and the invisible present: Memory, trauma, and representation in psychotherapy*. New York: Routledge.

Rizzolatti, G., Fogassi, L. & Gallese, V. (2006). Mirrors in the mind. *Scientific American*, November, 54–69.

Rutter, M. (1997). Clinical implications of attachment concepts: Retrospective and prospective. In L. Atkinson & K. J. Zucker (eds), *Attachment psychopathology* (pp. 17–46). New York: Guilford Press.

Schacter, D. L. (1987). Implicit memory: History and current status. *Journal of Experimental Psychology: Learning, Memory, and Cognition*, 13, 501–518.

Schacter, D. L. (1996). *Searching for memory: The brain, the mind, and the past*. New York: Basic Books.

Schore, A. N. (1994). *Affect regulation and the origin of the self: The neurobiology of emotional development*. Hillsdale, NJ: Lawrence Erlbaum Associates.

Schore, A. N. (2001). The effects of early relational trauma on right brain development, affect regulation, and infant mental health. *Infant Mental Health Journal*, 22, 201–269.

Schore, A. N. (2011). The right brain implicit self lies at the core of psychoanalysis. *Psychoanalytic Dialogues*, 21, 75–100.

Settlage, C. F., Rosenthal, J., Spielman, P. M., Gassner, S., Afterman, J., Bemesderfer, S. & Kolodny, S. (1990). An exploratory study of mother–child interaction during the second year of life. *Journal of the American Psychoanalytic Association*, 38, 705–731.

Shai, D. & Belsky, J. (2011). When words just won't do: Introducing parental embodied mentalizing. *SRCD Social Policy Report*, 5(3), 173–180.

Siegel, D. J. (2001). Toward an interpersonal neurobiology of the developing mind: Attachment relationships, "mindsight" and neural integration. *Infant Mental Health Journal*, 22, 67–94.

Siegel, D. J. (2012) *The Developing Mind: How relationships and the brain interact to shape who we are* (2nd edn). New York: Guilford Press.

Slade, A. (2004). The move from categories to process: Attachment phenomena and clinical evaluation. *Infant Mental Health Journal*, 25(4), 269–283.

Slade, A. (2005). Parental reflective functioning: An introduction. *Attachment & Human Development*, 7(3), 269–281.

Slade, A. (2008). Working with parents in child psychotherapy: Engaging the reflective function. In F. N. Busch (ed.), *Mentalization: Theoretical considerations, research findings, and clinical implications* (pp. 207–234). Hove: Analytic Press.

Slade, A. (2023). Looking back to light the path forward: Ghosts in the nursery revisited. *Infant Mental Health Journal*, 44(6), 857–868.

Sroufe, L. A. & Waters, E. (1977). Attachment as an organizational construct. *Child Development*, 48, 1184–1199.

Steele, H. & Steele, M. (2008). On the origins of reflective functioning. In F. N. Busch (ed.), *Mentalization: Theoretical considerations, research findings, and clinical implications* (pp. 133–158). New York: Analytic Press.

Stern, D. N. (1985). *The interpersonal world of the infant: A view from psychoanalysis and developmental psychology*. New York: Basic Books.

Stern, D. N., Sander, L. W., Nahum, J. P., Harrison, A. M., Lyons-Ruth, K., Morgan, A. C., Bruschweiler-Stern, N. & Tronick, E. Z. (1998). The process of therapeutic change involving implicit knowledge: Some implications of developmental observations for adult psychotherapy. *Infant Mental Health Journal*, 19(3), 300–308.

Szyf, M. and Bick, J. (2013). DNA methylation: A mechanism for embedding early life experiences in the genome. *Child Development*, 84(1), 49–57.

Teicholz, J. G. (2009). Introduction to "optimal responsiveness and the therapist's reaction to the patient's unresponsiveness". *Psychoanalytic Psychology*, 26(3), 235–238.

Tronick, E., Als, H., Adamson, L., Wise, S. & Brazelton, T. B. (1978). The infant's response to entrapment between contradictory messages in face-to-face interaction. *Journal of the American Academy of Child Psychiatry*, 17(1), 1–13.

Tronick, E. (2007). *The neurobehavioral and social-emotional development of infants and children*. New York: W. W. Norton.

Tyson, P. & Tyson, R. L. (1990). *Psychoanalytic theories of development: An integration*. New Haven: Yale University Press.

van der Kolk, B. A. (1994). The body keeps the score: Memory and the evolving psychobiology of post-traumatic stress. *Harvard Review of Psychiatry*, 1, 253–265.

van der Kolk, B. A. & Fisler, R. (1995). Dissociation and the fragmentary nature of traumatic memories: Overview and exploratory study. *Journal of Traumatic Stress*, 8(4), 505–521.

van der Kolk, B. A. (2005). Developmental trauma disorder: Towards a rational diagnosis for children with complex trauma histories. *Psychiatric Annals*, 35(5), 401–408.

van IJzendoorn, M. H. (1995). Adult attachment representations, parental responsiveness, and infant attachment: A meta-analysis on the predictive validity of the adult attachment interview. *Psychological Bulletin*, 117(3), 387–403.

van IJzendoorn, M. H. & Sagi, A. (1999). Cross-cultural patterns of attachment: Universal and contextual dimensions. In J. Cassidy & P. R. Shaver (eds), *Handbook of attachment: Theory, research, and clinical applications* (pp. 713–734). New York: Guilford Press.

van IJzendoorn, M. H. and Bakermans-Kranenburg, M. J. (2019). Bridges across the intergenerational transmission of attachment gap. *Current Opinion in Psychology*, 25, 31–36.

Wilkinson, M. (2010). *Changing minds in therapy: Emotion, attachment, trauma and neurobiology*. New York: Norton.

Winnicott, D. W. (1958). The capacity to be alone. *International Journal of Psychoanalysis*, 39, 416–420.

Winnicott, D. W. (1965). *The maturational processes and the facilitating environment: Studies in the theory of emotional development*. London: Hogarth Press.

Winnicott, D. W. (1974). Fear of breakdown. *International Journal of Psychoanalysis*, 55, 103–107.

Yehuda, R., Daskalakis, N. P., Bierer, L. M., Bader, H. N., Klengel, T., Holsboer, F. & Binder, E. B. (2016). Holocaust exposure induced intergenerational effects on FKBP5 methylation. *Biological Psychiatry*, 80(5), 372–380.

Zuckerman, M. (1998). Psychobiological theories of personality. In D. F. Barone, M. Hersen & V. B. Van Hasselt (eds), *Advanced personality* (pp. 123–154). New York: Plenum Press.

6 Memory, Trauma, and Representation in Psychotherapy

Retrospective Reflection

Stepping back from the argument developed in this chapter, what becomes most evident is how contemporary memory research reshapes the psychoanalytic landscape on which trauma, development, and therapeutic action have long been understood. The distinction between explicit and implicit memory systems does not merely supplement classical theory; it reorients it. Much of what psychoanalysis once sought to recover as repressed content now appears, in light of developmental neuroscience, as experience that was never symbolised to begin with – encoded procedurally, enacted relationally, and carried forward in the body as expectation rather than narrative.

This reframing brings the chapter into deep alignment with the volume's central thesis: that psychological life is fundamentally relational, co-constructed, and dynamically shaped by early patterns of attunement and disruption. Trauma, from this perspective, is not simply an event lodged in the past but an ongoing organisation of experience – a set of implicit dispositions that structure perception, affect, and relational possibility in the present. Dissociation, similarly, is understood not as a failure of will or insight but as a developmental and neurobiological disruption in the integration of memory systems, especially when early caregiving has been frightening, inconsistent, or absent. This formulation reflects the volume's wider concern with how psychological organisation emerges within intersubjective and developmental contexts.

Seen in this light, the therapeutic relationship becomes the primary site of transformation. It is within the immediacy of lived interaction – in the rhythms of attunement, rupture, and repair – that implicit relational patterns are activated, recognised, and gradually reorganised. These moments of procedural change shape the experiential substrate upon which reflective understanding can later be built. Insight, while valuable, is insufficient without this deeper re-patterning of implicit systems; yet explicit meaning-making remains essential for consolidating new possibilities for self-experience. Therapeutic action thus emerges as a dual process, enacted and articulated, embodied and symbolised.

DOI: 10.4324/9781003789727-9

This chapter also gestures forward, preparing the ground for later discussions in the volume that explore how clinicians work at the interface of these systems – how they listen not only to what is said but to what is enacted, how they track shifts in affective tone and bodily state, and how they participate in co-creating conditions in which previously unformulated experience can be felt, recognised, and eventually represented. The neurobiological emphasis on plasticity offers both hope and humility: change is possible, but it is neither instantaneous nor absolute. Trauma is not erased; rather, its activation becomes more recognisable, more tolerable, and more open to modulation within a relational field that can hold it.

In this sense, the chapter crystallises a theme that runs throughout the book: that the past lives on not as a fixed archive but as a dynamic set of relational and procedural tendencies, continually revised in the presence of another mind. Psychotherapy, at its best, provides a space in which these tendencies can be met, understood, and gradually transformed. The work is both subtle and profound – a process of reweaving implicit and explicit strands of experience into a more coherent, flexible, and compassionate sense of self. Later chapters take up this question more explicitly, examining how clinicians work moment-to-moment with enactment, affective shift, and bodily response as sites of therapeutic action.

Introduction

Recent developments in attachment research, trauma studies, and neuroscience have converged on a view of memory that has significant implications for psychoanalytic theory and practice. These developments challenge earlier clinical models that privileged verbal interpretation and the recovery of repressed content, suggesting instead that much of what organises experience and behaviour operates outside conscious awareness, is enacted rather than remembered, and is rooted in bodily and relational processes established early in development. From this perspective, therapeutic change cannot be understood solely in terms of insight or narrative reconstruction, but must also be conceived as a process that involves modification of implicit, procedural patterns of relating. It follows that, if cumulative trauma is encoded procedurally and transmitted implicitly, we must examine the memory systems through which this occurs. The concept of cumulative trauma, introduced earlier in the volume and elaborated in Chapter 5, provides a developmental and relational framework for understanding how such procedurally encoded experience is formed and transmitted.

This chapter brings together psychoanalytic theory and contemporary memory research to explicate the distinction between explicit (declarative) and implicit (non-declarative) memory systems, and to explore their relevance for understanding trauma, dissociation, and therapeutic action. I argue that traumatic experience, particularly when occurring in early attachment relationships, is often encoded in implicit memory systems that operate independently of autobiographical recall. As a consequence, such experience is not readily accessible to conscious remembering, but continues to shape perception, affect regulation, bodily states, and relational expectations in the present. Trauma, in this sense, is carried forward not primarily as a story that can be told, but as a way of being with oneself and others.

A central theme of the chapter is the idea that memory is not a static archive of past events, but a dynamic, reconstructive process that is continually revised in light of ongoing experience. This view resonates with Freud's early insight that we may not possess memories of childhood so much as memories relating to childhood (Freud, 1914), and with his emphasis on repetition as a form of remembering (Freud, 1920). Contemporary neuroscience has provided a complementary account of this phenomenon, demonstrating that memory is supported by multiple, partially independent systems, each with its own mode of encoding and retrieval (Schacter, 1996). Explicit memory allows for reflective recall and narrative organisation, whereas implicit memory is expressed through action, affect, and perception, often without awareness of its origins.

The implications of this distinction are particularly salient in the context of psychological trauma. Traumatic experience can overwhelm integrative mental processes and lead to dissociation, resulting in a fragmentation of experience across memory systems. In such circumstances, aspects of experience may be preserved as sensory impressions, emotional states, or procedural tendencies that are disconnected from explicit narrative meaning. These dissociated elements are frequently reactivated in situations that resemble earlier conditions of threat or misattunement, and may emerge in the therapeutic relationship as enactments rather than recollections. Understanding trauma in this way shifts the clinical focus from the recovery of forgotten events to the recognition and transformation of implicit patterns that organise experience in the present.

Within contemporary psychoanalysis, a range of concepts has been developed to describe forms of experience that are known without being symbolised, including unformulated experience (Stern, 1997), the unthought known (Bollas, 1987), implicit relational knowing (Boston Change Process Study Group, 2010; Lyons-Ruth et al., 1998), and fear of breakdown (Winnicott, 1974) that refer to events that have not yet been experienced as past. While differing in emphasis, these formulations converge on the idea that some aspects of experience are held outside reflective awareness and are communicated primarily through non-verbal and relational means. The present chapter situates these clinical observations within a broader framework provided by memory research, suggesting that they can be understood, at least in part, as manifestations of implicit memory processes.

The final aim of the chapter is to consider the role of explicit and implicit memory systems in therapeutic action. I argue that therapeutic change involves a dual process: the gradual modification of implicit, procedural patterns through lived relational experience, and the development of explicit understanding through reflection and meaning-making. These processes are mutually reinforcing and cannot be reduced to one another. From this perspective, the therapeutic relationship provides a context in which previously dissociated or unformulated experience can be enacted, recognised, and symbolised, allowing new forms of affect regulation and self-experience to emerge.

Comparison with Brewin's Dual Representation Theory

Before examining the explicit and implicit memory systems, it would be helpful to compare Brewin's dual representation theory with the relational-neurodevelopmental framework I am proposing.

From a cognitive psychology perspective, Brewin's dual representation theory (Brewin, Dalgleish & Joseph, 1996; Brewin, 2014, 2001) offers an important account of traumatic memory in terms of verbally accessible memory (VAM) and situationally accessible memory (SAM). This model helps to explain the persistence of sensory-affective fragments and intrusive re-experiencing in post-traumatic stress. Brewin's formulation is particularly illuminating in relation to discrete traumatic events and the failure to integrate them into autobiographical narrative.

The concept of cumulative relational trauma, however, operates at a different developmental level. Rather than addressing the fragmentation of a specific event, it concerns the gradual organisation of implicit relational systems within early attachment contexts. Here the issue is not primarily the persistence of intrusive memory, but the formation of procedural expectations – patterns of anticipation, affect regulation, and defensive organisation – that shape subsequent relational life. Such templates may precede the consolidation of episodic autobiographical memory altogether.

In this sense, the distinction is not oppositional but dimensional. Dual representation theory clarifies how traumatic events are stored and re-experienced; a relational-neurodevelopmental framework seeks to understand how chronic relational experience structures the developmental architecture within which later memories are encoded, interpreted, and enacted in relational encounters.

Memory Systems: Explicit and Implicit

This distinction becomes particularly salient in the clinical encounter, where patients may not re-experience discrete traumatic events as intrusive memories, but rather enact patterns of expectation, affect regulation, and relational anticipation whose origins lie beyond conscious recall. To understand how such patterns are retained and transmitted, it is necessary to consider contemporary accounts of memory organisation.

Research in cognitive neuroscience has demonstrated that memory is not a unitary faculty but comprises multiple, partially independent systems supported by distinct neural networks. Of particular relevance for psychoanalytic thinking is the distinction between explicit (declarative) and implicit (non-declarative) memory, as this provides a framework for understanding how relational experience may be encoded, expressed, and modified in the absence of conscious recollection.

Explicit memory refers to forms of memory available to conscious awareness and verbal report. It includes episodic memory – the recollection of autobiographical events situated in time and place – and semantic memory, or general knowledge about the world. These systems mature relatively late in development and support reflective thought, narrative organisation, and the construction of a coherent personal history. Importantly, explicit memories are not fixed records but are reconstructed at each recall, shaped by subsequent experience, affective state, and contextual meaning (Schacter, 1996; Damasio, 2000).

Implicit memory, by contrast, operates outside conscious awareness and is expressed through action, affect, perception, and bodily states rather than through narrative recollection. It includes procedural memory for skills and habits, as well as emotional and relational forms of memory that shape how individuals anticipate, interpret, and respond to their environment. Implicit memory is automatic in operation, does not require deliberate retrieval, and is not accessible to introspection in the usual sense. Instead, it is revealed indirectly through recurring patterns of behaviour, affective response, and relational expectation.

A crucial developmental finding is that the neural systems supporting implicit memory are functional from birth, whereas those supporting explicit memory mature gradually over the early years of life. As a result, early experience is encoded predominantly in implicit form, long before autobiographical memory or symbolic representation becomes available. This has important implications for understanding the persistence of early relational experience, including trauma, which may continue to shape functioning across the lifespan despite the absence of conscious recollection.

From a neurobiological perspective, implicit memory systems are closely linked to affective and motivational processes and are particularly sensitive to emotionally salient experience. When experience is characterised by intense arousal, threat, or relational misattunement, it may be encoded preferentially in these systems, especially where integrative capacities are compromised. Such memories are not forgotten but remain active as dispositions towards perception and action, shaping present experience without being recognised as originating in the past.

The distinction between explicit and implicit memory systems thus clarifies how experience may be both preserved and inaccessible – retained in action and affect without entering conscious narrative. It also allows classical psychoanalytic concerns with repetition and enactment to be reconsidered in developmental terms. What presents clinically as an inability to remember or to make use of insight may reflect the continued operation of implicit memory systems that function independently of conscious reflection, rather than repression in the traditional sense.

Within this perspective, trauma and dissociation can be understood not simply as the return of repressed content, but as disruptions in the integration of memory systems across development. Therapeutic action, accordingly, involves change at both implicit and explicit levels: the gradual reorganisation of procedural relational patterns alongside the emergence of reflective understanding.

Implicit Memory, the Unconscious, and Unformulated Experience

Across psychoanalytic traditions, clinicians have described forms of experience that are known without being symbolised, remembered without being consciously recalled, and expressed primarily through action, affect, and relational patterns. Concepts such as the unthought known (Bollas, 1987), unformulated experience (Stern, 1997), fear of breakdown (Winnicott, 1974), and implicit relational knowing (Boston Change Process Study Group, 2010; Lyons-Ruth et al., 1998) differ in emphasis, but converge on the idea that some aspects of experience are held outside reflective awareness and are not subject to repression in the classical sense. Rather, they arise from early developmental contexts in which the capacity for symbolic representation was not yet sufficiently established.

From the perspective of contemporary memory research, these clinical observations can be understood as manifestations of implicit or procedural memory processes. Experiences that occur prior to the maturation of explicit memory systems, or that overwhelm integrative capacities due to trauma, are encoded in non-declarative forms and retained as affective dispositions, bodily states, and relational expectations. Such experience is not forgotten, but remains active in shaping perception and behaviour, particularly in emotionally salient interpersonal contexts. Because these memories were never organised into narrative form, they cannot be retrieved through introspection alone, but must be accessed through their enactment in our relationships. The clinical implications of such disruptions for work with severe anxiety states and psychosis are taken up further in Chapter 12.

This understanding reframes classical psychoanalytic concerns with repetition and enactment. What appears clinically as compulsive repetition or resistance to insight may reflect the operation of implicit memory systems that function independently of conscious intention. In this sense, enactments in the transference are not simply defensive manoeuvres, but expressions of procedural knowledge acquired in earlier relational contexts. They represent attempts to manage current experience using strategies that were once adaptive, even if they have since become constraining.

Within the therapeutic relationship, these implicit patterns become available for transformation precisely because they are enacted rather than remembered. Through lived interaction, including moments of attunement, misattunement, and repair, previously unformulated aspects of experience may begin to acquire symbolic representation. This process does not involve the recovery of lost memories, but the creation of new meanings and new relational possibilities in the present. From this perspective, psychoanalytic work facilitates the integration of implicit and explicit modes of experience, allowing what was previously lived but unrepresented to become available for reflection, regulation, and choice.

Trauma, Dissociation, and Fragmentation

Psychological trauma refers to experiences that overwhelm an individual's capacity to regulate affect, maintain a coherent sense of self, and integrate experience into meaningful mental representations. Traumatic events are typically accompanied by intense fear, helplessness, and threat to psychological or physical integrity, disrupting the processes through which experience is ordinarily organised and symbolised. Trauma is therefore less usefully understood in terms of the objective characteristics of an event than in terms of its subjective impact and the relational context in which it is experienced.

A central psychological response to trauma is dissociation. First systematically described by Pierre Janet (1889), dissociation involves a disruption in the integration of experience, such that aspects of perception, affect, bodily sensation, and memory become segregated from one another. Rather than being assimilated into an integrated narrative of self-experience, traumatic material may be preserved in fragmented form, expressed through sensory impressions, affective states, and behavioural enactments (van der Kolk & Fisler, 1995). Dissociation does not erase traumatic experience, but alters the way it is encoded and retrieved.

From the perspective of memory research, dissociation may be understood as a disruption in the coordination of explicit and implicit memory systems. Under conditions of extreme arousal, integrative functions associated with reflective awareness and narrative organisation may be compromised, while systems involved in affective and procedural encoding remain active. As a result, traumatic experience is encoded predominantly in implicit forms, outside conscious recall, and later reactivated automatically in situations that resemble earlier conditions of threat or misattunement. Such reactivation is often experienced as occurring in the present rather than as a memory of the past.

Developmental research has highlighted the particular vulnerability of early experience to such processes. In infancy and early childhood, when explicit memory systems are immature, experience is encoded primarily in implicit, non-symbolic forms. Traumatic experience occurring within early attachment relationships may therefore have enduring effects on affect regulation, bodily states, and relational expectations, even in the absence of conscious memory. Importantly, it is often the cumulative impact of subtle, repeated disruptions in caregiver responsiveness, rather than discrete traumatic events, that leads to disorganisation and fragmentation of experience.

These findings help to explain why traumatic experience so frequently re-emerges in relational contexts, including psychotherapy, as enactment rather than recollection. Individuals may find themselves responding to present situations with intense affective reactions, bodily sensations, or expectations of danger or abandonment that appear disproportionate or inexplicable. Such responses reflect the activation of implicit memory systems shaped by earlier experience rather than failures of insight or resistance in the traditional sense.

Understanding trauma in this way shifts the clinical focus from the recovery of forgotten events to the recognition and transformation of implicit patterns that organise experience in the present. Therapeutic work involves attending to how traumatic experience is communicated through affect, bodily states, and relational dynamics, and creating conditions in which dissociated aspects of experience can be symbolised and integrated. This process depends less on reconstructing the past than on facilitating new forms of regulation, recognition, and meaning within the therapeutic relationship. How such implicit patterns emerge as enactments within the therapeutic relationship, and how clinicians work with them moment-to-moment, is examined in detail in Chapter 10.

Attachment, Representation, and Implicit Relational Memory

Early relationships play a central role in shaping the implicit organisation of experience. Attachment research has demonstrated that repeated patterns of interaction with caregivers give rise to internal working models (Bowlby, 1998, 1988) that structure expectations of self and other. These representational models are not primarily encoded as explicit beliefs or narratives, but as procedural forms of knowing that guide perception, affect regulation, and relational behaviour outside conscious awareness.

From a developmental perspective, the infant's capacity to regulate affect depends initially on the caregiver's responsiveness. Through repeated experiences of attunement, misattunement, and repair, the child internalises expectations about the availability and reliability of others, as well as about the manageability of internal states. When caregiving is sufficiently consistent and responsive, these implicit models support flexibility and resilience. When caregiving is frightening, withdrawn, or chronically misattuned, the resulting models may constrain experience and contribute to vulnerability to dissociation and affect dysregulation.

These representational models persist into adulthood as implicit relational expectations that shape interpersonal experience. Because they operate procedurally rather than reflectively, they are most readily accessed in the context of emotionally significant relationships, including psychotherapy. In this sense, transference may be understood as the activation of implicit relational memory rather than the displacement of specific remembered events. The therapeutic relationship thus becomes a primary site in which these models are enacted and potentially transformed.

The Role of Explicit and Implicit Memory in Therapeutic Action

From this perspective, therapeutic action does not consist primarily in the recovery of historically accurate memories, but in the gradual modification of implicit procedural patterns through which experience is organised and enacted in the present. Traumatic experience, particularly when occurring early in development, is encoded predominantly in non-declarative memory systems and expressed through affective states, bodily responses, and relational expectations rather than narrative recall.

Change occurs through a dual process (Boston Change Process Study Group, 2008). At the implicit level, new relational experiences within the therapeutic relationship allow alternative patterns of affect regulation and responsiveness to be enacted and encoded. At the explicit level, reflection and meaning-making supports the integration of these experiences into a more coherent sense of self. These processes are mutually reinforcing: implicit change provides the experiential foundation for reflection, while explicit understanding enhances flexibility and choice.

The therapeutic relationship is central to this process. Through repeated experiences of recognition, misattunement, and repair, previously dissociated or unformulated aspects of experience may become symbolised and integrated. This does not involve the erasure of traumatic memory, but the development of greater capacity to recognise and regulate its activation. In this sense, therapeutic action consists in expanding the individual's repertoire of responses, allowing movement between states of mind rather than entrapment within them.

Conclusion

This chapter has explored the relevance of contemporary understandings of memory for psychoanalytic thinking about trauma, dissociation, and therapeutic action. Central to this exploration has been the distinction between explicit and implicit memory systems, and the recognition that much of what organises experience, particularly following trauma, operates outside conscious awareness and is expressed through affective, bodily, and relational processes rather than narrative recall. From this perspective, traumatic experience is not simply something that happened in the past, but a mode of organisation that continues to shape perception, expectation, and behaviour in the present.

An appreciation of the dynamic and reconstructive nature of memory challenges models of therapeutic change that prioritise the recovery of forgotten events or the achievement of insight alone. While explicit reflection and meaning-making remain important, they are insufficient in the absence of changes at the level of implicit, procedural organisation. Traumatic experience, especially when embedded in early attachment relationships, is often encoded in forms that cannot be directly remembered, yet nevertheless exert a powerful influence through enactment and repetition. Therapeutic work must therefore attend to the ways in which such experience is lived and communicated within the relational field of treatment.

At the same time, contemporary findings on neural plasticity caution against both therapeutic omnipotence and therapeutic pessimism. While new experiences can lead to enduring changes in neural organisation and relational expectation, traumatic memories are not erased by treatment and may be reactivated in conditions of stress or loss. In this more modest sense, the aim of psychotherapy is not the elimination of trauma, but the development of greater capacity for affect regulation, reflective awareness, and flexibility in responding to internal and external experience.

From an intersubjective and psychodynamic perspective, the therapeutic relationship provides a unique context in which implicit patterns of relating can be enacted, recognised, and gradually transformed. Through repeated experiences of responsiveness, misattunement, and repair, previously dissociated or unformulated aspects of experience may become symbolised and integrated, allowing new representational models of self and other to emerge. In this way, therapeutic action can be understood as a dual process, involving both implicit change that is enacted within the relationship, and explicit change articulated through reflection and narrative. An integrated understanding of memory systems thus offers a framework for appreciating both the persistence of traumatic experience and the conditions under which meaningful psychological change can occur. These neurodevelopmental considerations are not abstract findings but become visible in the immediacy of the clinical encounter.

The next chapter revisits a classic psychoanalytic text – Klein's case study of Richard – through the lens of implicit memory and cumulative trauma, illustrating how these processes shape internal worlds.

References

Bollas, C. (1987). *The shadow of the object: Psychoanalysis of the unthought known*. London: Free Association Books.

Boston Change Process Study Group. (2008). Forms of relational meaning: Issues in the relations between the implicit and reflective-verbal domains. *Psychoanalytic Dialogues*, 18, 125–148.

Boston Change Process Study Group. (2010). *Change in psychotherapy: A unifying paradigm*. New York: Norton.

Bowlby, J. (1998). *Attachment and loss, vol. 2. Separation: Anxiety and Anger*. London: Pimlico.

Bowlby, J. (1988). *A secure base: Clinical applications of attachment theory*. London: Routledge.

Brewin, C. R. (2001). A cognitive neuroscience account of posttraumatic stress disorder and its treatment. *Behaviour Research and Therapy*, 39(4), 373–393.

Brewin, C. R. (2014). Episodic memory, perceptual memory, and their interaction: Foundations for a theory of posttraumatic stress disorder. *Psychological Bulletin*, 140(1), 69–97.

Brewin, C. R., Dalgleish, T. & Joseph, S. (1996). A dual representation theory of posttraumatic stress disorder. *Psychological Review*, 103(4), 670–686.

Damasio, A. (2000). *The feeling of what happens: Body, emotion and the making of consciousness*. London: Vintage.

Freud, S. (1914). Remembering, repeating and working-through. In J. Strachey (ed.), *The standard edition of the complete psychological works of Sigmund Freud*, vol. 12 (pp. 145–156). London: Hogarth Press.

Freud, S. (1920). Beyond the pleasure principle. In J. Strachey (ed.), *The standard edition of the complete psychological works of Sigmund Freud*, vol. 18 (pp. 7–64). London: Hogarth Press.

Freud, S. (1926). Inhibitions, symptoms and anxiety. In J. Strachey (ed.), *The standard edition of the complete psychological works of Sigmund Freud*, vol. 20 (pp. 77–174). London: Hogarth Press.

Janet, P. (1889). *L'automatisme psychologique: Essai de psychologie expérimentale sur les formes inférieures de l'activité humaine*. Paris: Félix Alcan.

Lyons-Ruth, K., Bruschweiler-Stern, N., Harrison, A. M., Morgan, A. C., Nahum, J. P., Sander, L. W., Stern, D. N. & Tronick, E. Z. (1998). Implicit relational knowing: Its role in development and psychoanalytic treatment. *Infant Mental Health Journal*, 19(3), 282–289.

Schacter, D. L. (1996). *Searching for memory: The brain, the mind, and the past*. New York: Basic Books.

Stern, D. B. (1997). *Unformulated experience: From dissociation to imagination in psychoanalysis*. Hillsdale, NJ: Analytic Press.

van der Kolk, B. A. & Fisler, R. (1995). Dissociation and the fragmentary nature of traumatic memories. *Journal of Traumatic Stress*, 8(4), 505–521.

Winnicott, D. W. (1974). Fear of breakdown. *International Journal of Psychoanalysis*, 1, 103–107.

7 Re-reading Klein

The Formation of Internal Worlds under Conditions of Cumulative Relational Trauma

Retrospective Reflection

Re-reading Klein's case study of Richard (Klein, 1945) through a contemporary relational lens invites a broader reflection on the evolution of psychoanalytic thought. Klein's clinical acuity remains astonishing; she saw into the child's symbolic world with a depth few have matched. Yet her theoretical commitments – particularly the primacy of innate aggression and the death instinct – constrained her ability to recognise the relational origins of the phenomena she so vividly described.

From today's vantage point, Richard's internal world appears less as a battleground of instinctual forces and more as a record of cumulative relational trauma. His persecutory anxieties, his oscillation between idealisation and fear, his phantasies of internal danger – all can be understood as the psychic imprint of a caregiving environment marked by depression, inconsistency, emotional silence, and repeated separations. This developmental reading extends the argument of Chapter 5, where early symbolic formations were shown to arise directly from relational patterns rather than instinctual imperatives.

This retrospective view does not diminish Klein's contribution. Rather, it reveals the generativity of her clinical material. Her observations continue to speak powerfully, but they speak differently when placed within a developmental, relational, and intergenerational frame. In this sense, Klein becomes not a figure to be corrected but a figure to be re-contextualised – a clinician whose insights remain fertile when read alongside contemporary understandings of attachment, trauma, and relational process.

Within the architecture of this book, this chapter serves as a hinge. It honours the depth of the psychoanalytic tradition while demonstrating how internal worlds are shaped by lived relational experience. It also prepares the ground for the chapters that follow, where the focus turns increasingly toward mentalisation and the therapeutic processes through which internal worlds can be transformed.

DOI: 10.4324/9781003789727-10

Introduction

This chapter builds on the developmental and relational foundations established in Chapters 5 and 6, using Klein's case of Richard to show how internal worlds are shaped by cumulative relational trauma rather than innate destructiveness. It also prepares the ground for Chapters 8–10, where issues of power, authority, mentalisation, and intergenerational transmission are explored. In this sense, the chapter functions as a hinge between the classical tradition and the relational-developmental arc of the book.

The chapter argues that Richard's internal world is best understood as the product of cumulative relational trauma rather than the inevitable expression of innate destructiveness. Klein's clinical observations remain vivid and clinically valuable, but when read through contemporary attachment and relational frameworks, the imagery of internal danger, fragmentation, and persecutory anxiety maps more directly onto a caregiving environment marked by parental depression, inconsistent availability, repeated separations, and unspoken family tensions (Bowlby, 1998).

A short vignette follows to anchor the chapter: A ten-year-old boy draws a house split down the middle, one side sunlit and the other partially erased, and says, "Sometimes it's like this, sometimes it's like that. I don't know which is real."

This image recurs throughout the chapter as a concrete illustration of how oscillating relational experience produces internal structures organised to survive instability. The chapter proceeds in four parts: the relational context and clinical material; the interpersonal mechanisms that shape internalisation; clinical technique and therapeutic change; and developmental and intergenerational implications.

Relational Context and Clinical Material

Richard's symptomatic world – persecutory anxieties, hypochondriasis, school refusal, clinging to mother, and fear of separations – aligns closely with patterns produced by anxious-insecure and disorganised attachment (Main & Hesse, 1990). The clinical history Klein recorded points repeatedly to relational conditions that generate such states: a mother described as depressed and inconsistently available, a father who was emotionally passive, repeated separations for hospitalisation and wartime evacuation, and a family culture of "no open trouble" in which conflict was present but unspoken.

These features create a caregiving environment in which emotional states are not named, contained, or shared. As Chapter 6 showed, when emotional life cannot be shared or spoken, the child's internal world becomes organised around threat, fragmentation, and the desperate search for stability. For a child exposed to such conditions, internal life becomes a record of relational experience: frightening parental affect is absorbed, separations are encoded as danger, and the absence of a regulating third leaves the mother-child dyad without a stabilising frame. Read this way, Richard's internal persecutors are not primarily expressions of innate aggression but adaptations to a relational world that repeatedly overwhelms his capacity for integration (Greenberg & Mitchell, 1988).

Klein records, for example, Richard's fear that bombs might enter his body and destroy him from within. She understood this as the projection of his own destructive impulses. Yet the imagery also belongs to a child living through wartime evacuation, parental anxiety, and repeated separations. External threat and internal fear converge. What appears as innate destructiveness can also be read as the psychic registration of an environment experienced as unpredictable, intrusive, and unprotected.

Mechanisms of Internalisation

Projective Identification as Two-Person Process

Projective identification functions here as an interpersonal exchange rather than a one-person intrapsychic process (Lyons-Ruth, 1999). The child projects unbearable affect into caregivers who, because of their own unprocessed states, respond in ways that confirm those projections. Over time, the child internalises these unmentalised states as persecutory objects.

In lived interaction, this process may be subtle but powerful. A child overwhelmed by anxiety may become restless or demanding; a depressed or emotionally preoccupied caregiver may withdraw, respond irritably, or fail to provide coherent reassurance (Green). The child then experiences the caregiver as rejecting or frightening, thereby confirming the very expectation that prompted the projection. What begins as an attempt to evacuate unmanageable affect crystallises into a relational pattern that stabilises persecutory internal figures.

Splitting as Trauma-Evoked Defence

Splitting preserves access to caregivers by separating their good and bad aspects into distinct internal objects. In contexts of inconsistent caregiving, splitting is a pragmatic defence: it allows the child to maintain hope for care while managing fear (Fonagy & Target, 2000). Richard's oscillation between idealisation and persecution of his mother mirrors the oscillation of caregivers' behaviour.

Role Reversal and the Parentified Child

When caregivers are depressed or overwhelmed, children often assume emotional caretaking roles. This "parentified child" stance sacrifices the child's developmental needs for exploration and regulation (Bowlby, 1998).

The burden of carrying a caregiver's unmentalised affect intensifies internal persecutory imagery and constrains opportunities for healthy differentiation, as explored in Chapter 2.

Failure of Triangulation

An emotionally absent father removes a crucial regulatory third. Without triangulation, the dyadic intensity between mother and child remains unmodulated, increasing the likelihood of disorganised attachment strategies and internal worlds organised around threat and fragmentation (Fonagy & Target, 1999). Without a stabilising third, the integration of ambivalence that characterises the depressive position remains precarious.

Clinical Technique and Therapeutic Change

Interpretation as Containment

Klein's direct interpretations can be reframed as early forms of affective naming. For a child whose family does not name or hold emotional states, the analyst's capacity to articulate internal experience provides corrective relational meaning. Interpretation functions as containment when it is offered within an attuned, contingent relationship. This anticipates the mentalisation-based processes explored in Part III, where containment becomes the foundation for reflective functioning and the emergence of new relational procedures.

From a relational perspective, such interpretation need not foreground the child's aggression. It may instead articulate the fear or instability that organises the aggression. An intervention might sound less like the exposure of a destructive wish and more like the naming of a precarious experience: "When everything feels as though it might fall apart, it can be frightening and lonely. I wonder if something like that is happening now." In this way, meaning is co-constructed rather than imposed, and affect becomes thinkable within the safety of relationship.

Reparation as Relational Stabilisation

Reparation, in this relational reading, is the child's attempt to stabilise precarious relationships rather than merely to atone for destructive impulses. Omnipotent phantasies of repair reflect a desperate effort to maintain connection with caregivers who feel fragile or inconsistent. Therapeutic reparation occurs when the analytic relationship offers reliable responsiveness that the family could not provide.

From One-Person to Two-Person Psychology

Klein's clinical acuity is preserved while expanding the explanatory frame to include the analyst's participation. A relational stance emphasises mutual influence, attunement, and repair. The analyst's interventions are most effective when they co-construct meaning with the child rather than impose interpretation from a solely intrapsychic model.

Developmental and Intergenerational Implications

Attachment continuity, reflective caregiving, and relational stability are prerequisites for the developmental achievement Klein called the depressive position – the capacity to hold ambivalence and integrate good and bad in the same object. When caregiving is fragmented, the movement towards integration is delayed or disrupted.

Family systems dynamics also matter. From this perspective, the child often functions as the "identified patient" who embodies unprocessed family conflict (Minuchin, 1974). Unspoken conflict and wartime anxieties transmit across generations when emotional states are not symbolised or mentalised. Therapeutic work therefore attends not only to the child's intrapsychic structures but to the relational patterns that sustain them. This intergenerational transmission sets the stage for the systemic patterns examined in Chapter 9, where family dynamics become the carriers of unprocessed affect.

Conclusion

Reframing Klein's case through attachment and relational lenses preserves her clinical observations while relocating their origins in lived relational experience. Richard's persecutory objects, splitting, and phantasies of internal danger emerge coherently from a caregiving environment marked by parental depression, inconsistent availability, repeated separations, emotional silence, and the absence of a regulating third. Therapeutic change follows from providing a relational context in which affect can be named, held, and repaired, enabling the child to move towards integration and a sense of felt security (Bowlby, 1998).

Ultimately, Richard's recovery suggests that the repair of such deep-seated persecutory anxieties requires more than the interpretation of phantasy; it necessitates the kind of sustained procedural transformation and "moments of meeting" that form the heart of the clinical encounter explored in Part III.

This relational re-reading does not negate Klein's insights; it re-contextualises them, showing how the same clinical material can illuminate both intrapsychic symbolism and the developmental consequences of cumulative relational trauma. The relational vulnerabilities traced here become the very material through which asymmetrical dynamics are enacted, both in families and in the consulting room.

The next chapter examines how power and authority shape these internal structures and their enactments in asymmetrical relationships, including the therapeutic setting itself. Within this reframing, the death instinct recedes as a primary explanatory principle and becomes instead a metaphor for the child's lived experience of relational collapse, fragmentation, and uncontained fear.

Like the boy who drew the house split down the middle, Richard's recovery depended on the gradual possibility of holding both sides of experience within a single, coherent frame.

References

Bowlby, J. (1998). *Attachment and loss, vol. 2. Separation: Anxiety and anger.* London: Pimlico.

Fonagy, P. & Target, M. (1999). Towards understanding violence: The use of the body and the role of the father. In R. S. Perelberg (ed.), *Psychoanalytic understanding of violence and suicide* (pp. 53–72). London: Routledge.

Fonagy, P. & Target, M. (2000). Playing with reality: III. The persistence of dual psychic reality in borderline patients. *International Journal of Psychoanalysis*, 81, 853–873.

Green, A. (1983). The dead mother. *International Journal of Psychoanalysis*, 64, 289–299.

Greenberg, J. R. & Mitchell, S. A. (1988). *Object relations in psychoanalysis.* Cambridge, MA: Harvard University Press.

Klein, M. (1945). The Oedipus complex in the light of early anxieties. In J. Steiner (ed.), *The Oedipus complex today* (pp. 3–30). London: Karnac Books.

Lyons-Ruth, K. (1999). The two-person unconscious: Intersubjective dialogue, enactive relational representation, and the emergence of new forms of relational organization. *Psychoanalytic Inquiry*, 19(4), 576–617.

Main, M. & Hesse, E. (1990). Parents' unresolved traumatic experiences are related to infant disorganized attachment status: Is frightened and/or frightening parental behavior the linking mechanism? In M. Greenberg, D. Cicchetti and E. M. Cummings (eds), *Attachment in the preschool years: Theory, research and intervention* (pp. 161–182). Chicago, IL: University of Chicago Press.

Minuchin, S. (1974). *Families and family therapy*. Cambridge, MA: Harvard University Press.

8 Power, Security, and Recognition

Attachment, Authority, and Relational Trauma

Retrospective Reflection

This chapter was written out of a growing concern with how experiences of power and powerlessness shape attachment, development, and later relational expectations. While much attachment-informed writing has focused on security, attunement, and regulation, less attention has been paid to the role of authority, asymmetry, and coercion in the organisation of the inner world. Returning to this chapter now, I see it as an early attempt to address that gap.

From the perspective developed across this volume, experiences of powerlessness may be understood as a central dimension of cumulative relational trauma. For children, caregivers inevitably occupy positions of authority, and when that authority is exercised in frightening, inconsistent, or coercive ways, the developing self may adapt through compliance, dissociation, or identification with the aggressor. These adaptations are not pathological in themselves, but they carry forward implicit expectations about relationships, safety, and recognition.

This chapter extends attachment theory into social, cultural, and political domains, drawing on psychoanalytic and social psychological perspectives to examine how authority and submission are internalised. Read alongside later chapters on enactment, sexuality, and violence, it can be seen as preparing the ground for understanding how power dynamics re-emerge within therapeutic relationships and other asymmetrical contexts. In this sense, the chapter functions as a bridge between developmental theory and the ethical complexities of relational clinical practice. It therefore extends the argument that internal worlds are shaped within asymmetrical relational systems whose exercise of authority may either facilitate integration or entrench trauma.

Introduction

In the previous chapter, I reconsidered the formation of internal worlds under conditions of cumulative relational trauma, suggesting that

DOI: 10.4324/9781003789727-11

persecutory anxieties and fragmentation are rooted not primarily in innate destructiveness but in lived experiences of instability, inconsistency, and uncontained affect. If internal structures emerge from relational conditions, then the organisation of power within those conditions becomes central. The child's experience of authority – whether benign, neglectful, frightening, or coercive – shapes not only attachment security but expectations about recognition, agency, and survival in asymmetrical relationships.

This chapter examines power as a central dimension of attachment, trauma, and therapeutic relationships. Power is an implicit thread in the discourses that inform many aspects of our social and political life. Power relations are rarely equal or symmetrical.

Indeed, it would seem to be an indisputable fact of social and political life that power relations are inherently asymmetrical, including, of course, the relationship between the therapist and the patient, notwithstanding the concept of mutual reciprocal influence (Aron, 1996). Frankel (2002) argues that the asymmetrical exercise of power is intrinsically traumatic because it induces fear of isolation and emotional abandonment.

Asymmetry in power relations gives rise to evaluative questions: is power being used in a benign, constructive way, or in a malign, harmful way? If the effect on the other is malignant, how witting or unwitting, explicit or implicit, conscious or unconscious are the processes involved? Moreover, what mental states underlie the abuse of power – fear, shame, hate? Sullivan (1953, 1962) argued that we are all involved in subtle and not so subtle "security operations" in our interpersonal lives wherein one person's sense of safety and security is established at the expense of the other person's. In extreme cases, as Searles (1993) and Laing and Esterson (1964) have shown, people in close relationships may use their greater power effectively to drive the other person crazy.

Socio-cultural Factors

At a societal level, we need to consider the impact of powerlessness on the mental health of persons from ethnic minorities who are alienated from the mainstream white culture by institutionalised racism. Extending Freud's (1917) theory of melancholia to the experience of Asian-Americans, Eng and Han (2001) argue that racial melancholia underpins everyday experiences of immigration, assimilation, racialisation, and group identity. In the therapeutic relationship, implicit and explicit power relations are likely to emerge into the foreground when the dyad consists of people who differ in terms of race, class, gender, and sexual orientation. The resulting struggle for domination, however subtle, may reflect historical inequalities and a legacy of denial of the other's subjectivity by those in power (Benjamin, 1988, 1995; Fletchman Smith, 2000; Mitchell & Black, 1996).

Following Ferenczi (1933), Frankel (2002) conceptualises this process in terms of a mutual identification with the aggressor, with each person vying to gain a sense of security by controlling the dangerous other. From this perspective, identification with the aggressor is directed towards undoing the sense of powerlessness and fear of abandonment that each partner in the dyad experiences, however unconsciously. This defence may also operate in everyday life in relation to those who have power and authority over us. In the therapeutic situation, we need to question to what extent we can tolerate difference, remain open to learning from the patient, and allow patients to impact on and transform us (Casement, 1990; Ghent, 1992).

On a wider stage, the power wielded by what may be termed sociopathic political leaders may be seen in various international settings. Often there appears to be a passive collusion by the population with a mad, socio-political "reality". These dynamics may be paralleled in the power relations operating in the country's social systems, including family systems. Miller (1991) roots tyrannical leaders' abuse of power in their traumatic childhoods, arguing that their political careers are governed by the idea of "redemption through destruction" (p. 105). Accepting that the meaning of behaviour is, in part, culturally organised and mediated, Miller's (1991) studies of tyrannical leaders emphasise the need to consider how the wider socio-political context interacts with psychological development; how, as therapists, our internalisation of, and identification with, external power structures and cultural institutions may influence the therapeutic relationship.

The Agentic Self

Milgram (1974) draws a distinction between an autonomous mode of functioning and an agentic state. The shift from self-agency to the agentic state is triggered by the act of defining a person of higher social status as part of an authority system of relevance to the subject. An authority system consists of a minimum of two persons sharing the expectation that one of them has the right to prescribe behaviour for the other. He found that there is a transition from the moment when the person stands outside an authority system to the moment when they are inside it. This may include crossing a physical threshold into the authority figure's domain. Entry into the authority figure's realm of authority is voluntarily undertaken. The psychological consequence of this is that it creates a sense of commitment and obligation which binds the subject to their role in the process.

There is general agreement not only that the authority figure can influence behaviour but that they ought to be able to do so. Thus, power comes about in some degree through the consent of the person over whom the authority figure presides. As Milgram (1974) emphasises, once the subject grants this consent, its withdrawal proceeds at great social cost. In the light of these findings, it may be accepted that the potential for the abuse of power in the therapeutic situation is substantial.

Such social and relational dynamics may also be seen in patriarchy, a hierarchical system characterised by male domination and female subordination. Feminists argue that patriarchy is such a powerful ideology that men are usually able to secure the apparent voluntary consent of the very women they oppress. Such domination often takes the form of sexual harassment and sexual assault. In recent years, the "MeToo" movement was founded to raise awareness of the prevalence and pernicious impact of sexual violence perpetrated by men against vulnerable women and to empower survivors of such violence and unequal power relations.

These dynamics of domination, misrecognition, and the collapse of agency are not confined to large-scale social structures; they are lived out in intimate relationships where attachment fear and power asymmetry become tightly intertwined. Hardeep's history offers a stark illustration of how coercive control may emerge from an unresolved and disorganised attachment system rather than from conscious malice or entitlement.

Following the death of his father, Hardeep became the emotional centre of gravity for his anxious, dependent mother. Her grief and fear bound him into an inverted caregiving role, leaving him developmentally overburdened and unable to differentiate his own needs from hers. Attempts to assert autonomy were met with guilt, anxiety, and subtle coercion, creating a relational template in which proximity was maintained through emotional pressure rather than mutual recognition. The absence of a stabilising third left the dyad without symbolic space, intensifying the fusion of fear and responsibility that Chapter 7 described as fertile ground for disorganisation.

When his partner, Jaswinder, attempted to end their relationship, these early relational patterns were reactivated with overwhelming force. Her withdrawal triggered a collapse of his fragile regulatory capacities, activating what Liotti (1992) describes as a multiple, incoherent representational model. Hardeep oscillated between clinging dependency and coercive control, seeking proximity through intrusive contact, surveillance, and ultimately violence. His behaviour, while destructive, can be understood as a desperate attempt to restore attachment security in the face of unbearable fear, shame, and the threat of psychic annihilation. In such moments, recognition collapses: the other ceases to exist as a separate subject and is instead experienced as the bearer of the self's survival.

Seen through this lens, Hardeep's actions represent a pathological form of attachment behaviour – "attachment gone wrong" (de Zulueta, 1993) – in which coercion becomes a maladaptive strategy for containing dysregulated affect and warding off the terror of abandonment.

Power and Intersubjectivity

Exploring further the issue of power in the therapeutic setting, relational and intersubjective theorists such as Mitchell (1993, 1997; Mitchell & Black, 1996) and Benjamin (1988, 1995) argue that there has been a paradigm shift from a one-person, drive theory model to a two-person, relational model. This has led to a concomitant shift in the role of the analyst from that of a neutral, anonymous all-knowing expert to that of an active co-participant whose countertransference provides an important source of information about both their own and the patient's subjective experience. From this perspective, intersubjectivity refers to our experience of the other as separate and having an equivalent centre of self. A shared reality comes to be established by means of a subtle intertwining of both intrapsychic and interpersonal processes (Benjamin, 1995). Thus, psychological meaning is negotiated and co-constructed in the here-and-now through interaction in the intersubjective field rather than regarded as being universal and biologically inherent, as in drive theory (Mitchell, 1993).

In terms of power, the relational analyst openly acknowledges that their theories, patterns of thought, and systems of ideas have an important influence on the therapeutic process. Indeed, the personal attributes of the analyst are viewed as playing a significant part in organising and integrating the patient's material, thereby providing shape and structure to their inner world (Mitchell, 1993; Mitchell & Black, 1996). It is also assumed that this process is mutual and that the patient will change the therapist as part of a continuous process of bi-directional influence in the intersubjective field (Aron, 1996).

An interactional conceptualisation of the therapeutic process is consistent with the findings of infant research (Beebe & Lachmann, 1992, 2002). This challenges the view of countertransference as a static, intermittent event occurring in reaction to the patient's transference. Mutual reciprocal influence, however, does not imply equal influence, in that the relationship can be mutual without being symmetrical (Aron, 1996). The therapist's struggle to understand and recover from "mistakes" and re-enactments without becoming defensive or inauthentic is seen as a central aspect of the therapeutic relationship, leading to mutual recognition and change (Aron, 1996; Frankel, 2002; Mitchell, 2000). Mitchell (1993) compares this model to that employed by Freud (1905) in his brief analysis of Dora. Despite Freud (1905) being fully aware that Dora had been profoundly betrayed by those she most trusted, his theoretical frame led him to focus on intrapsychic neurotic conflict, thereby invalidating her subjective experience and perpetuating, in the countertransference, her victimisation by the men in her life.

Frankel (2002), however, notes that no technique can eliminate the inherent power differential in the therapeutic relationship, or the therapist's unconscious use of this relationship for good or for ill. Mann (1997) argues that the therapist's open recognition of their erotic desire and subjectivity indicates a mature awareness of the differentiation between self and other which may help to preclude the sexual abuse of the patient. However, he cautions against disclosing such erotic feelings to the patient.

By contrast, Aron (1996) advocates allowing the patient access to the therapist's subjectivity, in terms of disclosing their thoughts, feelings, and fantasies. He argues that this leads to an acknowledgement by the patient of the therapist as a separate subject. This intersubjective aspect of the therapeutic process may protect the patient from passively complying with, and submitting to, the therapist's power and authority. More generally, Aron (1996) and Benjamin (1992) point out that an awareness of the way in which our own subjectivities and theoretical orientation influences and limits the multiple possibilities of the therapeutic relationship merely raises new problems of power, in terms of a tension between mutuality and asymmetry, together with thorny questions about what the analyst knows and does not know.

In discussing "knowledge as power", Benjamin (1992) cautions against idealising a stance of not-knowing in reaction to the old classical ideal of analytic certitude. Indeed, Winnicott, in his final paper, contends that the therapist can hold up the patient's progress "because of genuinely not knowing". For example, he argues that the patient's "clinical fear" of a future breakdown is, in fact, the fear of a breakdown that has already happened but which has "not yet been experienced". He suggests that the patient needs to be told about this crucial aspect of their experience (Winnicott, 1974, pp. 176–177).

Disclosure of the kind advocated by Winnicott (1974) may be seen as prefiguring the intersubjective technique of selectively revealing the therapist's subjectivity. In this context, Frankel (2006) acknowledges the reluctance in contemporary psychoanalytic circles to diagnose the patient out of fear that this kind of "knowing" may negate or obliterate the patient's subjective experience. This notwithstanding, he argues that diagnosis is an idea that cannot easily be given up because people do have distinctive personality characteristics and limitations that endure over time. He posits a relational model that includes the concept of "diagnosis-of-the-moment": an interactive process that informs how the therapist responds moment-by-moment to the patient's changing self-states and multiple ways of organising experience.

For their part, Aron and Anderson (1998) emphasise the way in which what the therapist knows is informed by their observations of the patient's body, in terms of gesture, facial display, and posture. Similarly, Orbach (1995, 1999, 2004) highlights the use of the therapist's body countertranference to register and understand the patient's implicit affective states and communication of unconscious material.

Developmental Issues

Influenced by Winnicott (1960) and the findings of more recent empirical developmental studies by Stern (1985) and Beebe and Lachmann (1992), Mitchell (1993) argues that deficiencies in caregiving in the earliest years interfere with the emergence of a fully centred and integrated sense of self and the development of subjectivity. He suggests that in many respects the "good enough" caregiver-infant relationship constitutes the prototype of a therapeutic model in work with adults – that the analytic process is redolent of the subtle intersubjective, communicative, and regulatory processes that take place between the caregiver and the child.

From a relational perspective, the inner world is viewed as developing through these mutually reciprocal influences, and the mind as being composed of relational configurations developed in interaction with others. Similarly, Fonagy (1999a) argues that the child's experience of self becomes meaningful in the context of the caregiver's response to their expressions of psychological states. When this intersubjective process is less than optimal because of the abuse of power in the child-parent relationship, the transmission of trauma across generations (Fonagy, 1999a; Holmes, 1999; Peck, 2003), or the parent's compromised capacity for mentalisation (Bateman & Fonagy, 2004; Fonagy et al., 1995; Slade, 2005), the child may identify with the aggressor (Ferenczi, 1933; A. Freud, 1993) and develop a false self (Winnicott, 1960).

Anna Freud's (1993) conceptualisation of identification with the aggressor differs from Ferenczi's earlier formulation in significant ways. She views identification with the aggressor as a defensive process whereby children transform themselves "from the person threatened into the person who makes the threat" (p. 113). For Anna Freud, the change from the passive role to the active role is a means of assimilating "dissociated" traumatic experience which is turned into "an active assault on the outside world" (p. 116).

By contrast, Ferenczi (1933), based on his work with adult survivors of childhood sexual abuse, argues that identification with the aggressor is a response to an overwhelming threat in situations where there is no physical escape. The abused, helpless child becomes oblivious of themselves, identifying with the menacing aggressor and passively gratifying their desires. In subordinating themselves to the aggressor, the child disappears, being transformed into the image that the aggressor has of them. As Frankel (2002) notes, both forms of identification with the aggressor may be in operation simultaneously, being used to adapt to a threatening external reality, as well as to cope with disturbing inner feelings that arise as a result of a threat to the self.

Ferenczi's (1933) concept addresses similar issues to Winnicott's (1960) "false self" organisation. This defensive structure comprises a compliant, acquiescent way of organising self-experience in reaction to developmental conflict in the infant-caregiver relationship (Mills, 2003). In such instances, the child withdraws from self-generated spontaneity and instead conforms to the imposed images and needs of the caregiver upon whom they depend for love, protection, and security. In suppressing vital aspects of self-experience, the child adopts an alien reality and inauthentic mode of being and relating (Mills, 2003). Winnicott (1967) contends that, in a phenomenological sense, the child ceases to exist in those moments when the parent fails to greet their spontaneous gesture. Moreover, he argues that the caregiver's failure to mirror the child's current state leads to an internalisation of the caregiver's actual state, which then becomes an alien part of the child's nascent self-structure (Winnicott, 1967).

In a relationship with a caregiver who is frightened and/or frightening, either because of suffering unresolved trauma and entering dissociative states, or because of being actively abusive, the child incorporates the parent's feelings of rage, hate, and fear, together with an image of themselves as toxic and frightening. "This image must then be externalised for the child to achieve a bearable and coherent self-representation" (Fonagy, 1999b, p. 103). Lacking a coherent, organised strategy for coping with the stress of separation, the child regulates their fear by becoming increasingly aggressive and controlling (Hesse & Main, 2000; Lyons-Ruth & Jacobvitz, 1999; Solomon, et al., 1995). If unresolved, this parent-child controlling relational dynamic is carried into adulthood and enacted in the person's intimate relationships, particularly in contexts involving separation and loss (Renn, 2003, 2006, 2007).

From a Winnicottian perspective, the insecurely attached child develops a "false self", which functions as a "caretaker self" to protect the potential "true self" (Winnicott, 1960, p. 142). The prevalence of the "false self" phenomenon in contemporary society, in the form of obdurate, merged attachments to internalised inauthentic and constricted relational configurations, has led Mitchell (1993) to assert that pseudo-normality is the clinical problem of our time.

Aggression, Maternal Subjectivity, and Mutual Recognition

To balance these views, Kraemer (1996) argues that Winnicott (1947) does not sufficiently address the discomfort normative hate can generate in the mother, or the conflict the mother feels in owning her desire for power and control. Kraemer (1996) points out that, in using a developmental model in work with adults, consideration of the mother's subjectivity is largely absent or ignored. Just as the therapist's experience of herself and her patient is now increasingly recognised, Kraemer (1996) argues that there is a need to recognise the complexity and ambivalence of the mother's reactions to her baby's affective communications, including multiple and oscillating self-states and a confused sense of power and powerlessness. She suggests that fear of exploiting and abusing the baby may direct the mother away from acknowledging more fully how much she needs the baby to meet her own needs and desires. Kraemer (1996) contends that similar power dynamics may be enacted between analyst and patient in the therapeutic relationship.

In this context, Benjamin (1995) questions to what extent any aspect of subjectivity may be privileged as the truer, authentic part in relation to which other parts are false or inauthentic. However, influenced by Winnicott (1947, 1960, 1971), she amplifies Mahler et al.'s (1985) theory of separation-individuation, stressing the role that aggression plays in the development of intersubjectivity.

Benjamin (1995) argues that mutual recognition and intersubjective relatedness are not inevitable aspects of infant development but rather are developmental achievements. The parent-infant relationship may either be oppressive and controlling or facilitating and liberating. The struggle for recognition brings forth aggression and thus separation which fosters a symbolic space between mother and child. Benjamin (1995) sees this developmental process as the necessary basis for non-coercive intersubjectivity, noting that relatedness is characterised not by continuous harmony but by continuous disruption and repair (Beebe & Lachmann, 1992). When the process of mutual recognition breaks down because of conflict in the mother-infant relationship, experience is organised predominantly intrapsychically rather than intersubjectively, the upshot of which is a struggle for power (Benjamin, 1995).

Separation, Identity, and the Role of Trauma

Mitchell's (1993) theoretical position, as summarised above, resonates with the respective ideas of McDougall (1990), Bollas (1987) and, in particular, Fairbairn (1952). These theorists argue that all psychopathological developments in the adult are based on a failure to attain psychological differentiation. Fairbairn (1952) views the failure of this developmental accomplishment as deriving from feelings of insecurity stemming from separation anxiety. Authors as diverse as Khan (1979), McDougall (1990), Schore (1991, 1994, 2001) and van der Kolk (1989, 1994) view the persistence of a disturbed form of child-parent interaction as constituting cumulative trauma.

Influenced by Mahler et al., (1985), Stoller (1986) and Stubrin (1994) contend that the mother's inability to facilitate the child's separation and psychological differentiation results in self-alienation and identity diffusion, particularly in a relational matrix in which the father is weak, powerless, or absent. These authors view such relational dynamics as linked to a form of adult psychopathology in which dissociated hatred and hostility are acted out in perverse or neo-sexual ways, arguing that the primary motivation for such activity is the desire to separate and form a distinct identity.

The role of the father in helping the child to separate from a disturbed relationship with the mother is seen as a vital aspect of the child's relational experience (Campbell, 1999; Khan, 1979). Indeed, Fonagy and Target (1999) argue that the perspective of the father as a third object may provide the child with a second chance to develop a secure psychological self. In line with Stoller (1986), Litowitz (2002) contends that non-sexual defensive motivation may take on a sexualised nature when the person's sense of self is endangered and under threat. Frankel (2002) argues that identification with the aggressor is a widespread phenomenon and one that is by no means restricted to people who have suffered severe trauma. He concludes that "some degree or element of trauma has played an important role in the lives of many people in whose histories trauma does not appear prominent" (p. 117).

The prevalence of more overt forms of malignant parental power, in the form of neglect and sexual, emotional, and physical abuse, has been comprehensively documented in the abuse and trauma literature. For example, Davies and Frawley (1994) and Bromberg (1998) have shown how a relational matrix characterised by abuse can lead to the development of multiple self-states. Here, traumatic experience is dissociated and encapsulated within the personality as a separate, non-reflective reality cut off from authentic human relatedness.

Fonagy (1999a) contends that unresolved trauma destroys the capacity to reflect on and appraise the mental states that give meaning to subjective experience and social behaviour. Davies (2004) argues that in work with survivors of sexual abuse, the therapist is required to make multiple shifting diagnoses in response both to the vicissitudes of the patient's self-states and to the different roles that therapists themselves are drawn into enacting in the transference-countertransference matrix. In this context, it needs to be kept in mind that powerlessness is a key feature of trauma, and that dissociation in reaction to trauma walls off access to self-experience and emotional connection with others.

Power, Intersubjectivity, and the Role of Security

As Frankel (2002) emphasises, the work of Bowlby (1997, 1998a, 1998b), Fairbairn (1952) and Sullivan (1953, 1962) suggests that our most basic need is attachment. Given this, I would argue that security is more salient and significant than aggression in promoting non-defensive separation and psychological differentiation, thereby facilitating the child's innate potential for mutual recognition and intersubjective relatedness. While normative levels of aggression may promote autonomy and independence, uncontained or disavowed aggressive behaviour may be seen as motivated by fear, shame, rage, and hate. Such negative affective states are contained and tempered by a consistent and reliable process of interactive regulation and the repair of inevitable disruptions in the child-parent relationship (Beebe & Lachmann, 1992, 2002; Schore, 1991, 1994, 2001).

Infancy research indicates that it is this intersubjective process, together with the parent's capacity for reflective functioning, which promotes security. This enables the child to regulate the tension between attachment and separation and thus explore their own mind in relation to the minds of others as a differentiated psychological self (Fonagy & Target, 2005; Grienenberger, et al., 2005; Slade, 2005). In reconsidering Mahler et al.'s (1985) theory, Lyons-Ruth (1991) suggests that the first two years of life should be reframed from a separation-individuation process to an attachment-individuation process.

The lack of an internal sense of security deriving from the breakdown of attachment processes constitutes cumulative relational trauma. The child whose subjective experience has consistently been negated or obliterated is likely to defensively avoid knowing the thoughts and feelings in the mind of the other for fear of discovering a hostile or malevolent intent or, more frightening still, as not existing at all (Fonagy et al., 1995; Knox, 2001, 2003). As Fonagy (1999b) and Holmes (1999) argue, the parent's unresolved traumatic and fearful states of mind can be transmitted to the child, leading to states of disorganisation and dissociation, even though they have not been directly abused or traumatised. Thus, social referencing and the sharing of differentiated emotional states, key aspects of intersubjective relatedness, are precluded (Stern, 1985). In a relational matrix such as this, the child's capacity to be alone – to forget the mother in the confident expectation that she will be available when remembered – fails to develop (Winnicott, 1958). The consequent hyper-vigilant need to monitor and adapt to the other's affective states leads to a confusion of self with other (Ferenczi, 1933).

Conclusion

In my view, developmental experiences of the kinds outlined above account for the frequency of Frankel's (2002) clinical experience relating to the role of trauma, Winnicott's (1974) clinical finding of a widespread fear of breakdown, and Fairbairn's (1952) theory that the revival of traumatic scenes re-traumatises the person. Clinically, such early preverbal phenomenological experience appears to consist of implicitly encoded emotional memories (Orange, 1995; Schacter, 1996) imbued with a pervasive sense of fear and dread – what Winnicott (1974) termed "primitive agonies" and Bion (1984) called "nameless dread".

In terms of Bion's (1984) theory, the caregiver has not been able to enter a requisite state of reverie to contain, transform, and give meaning to the infant's inchoate anxiety and terror. The inability to symbolically represent and reflect on traumatic states of mind motivates a controlling attitude to self and other in later life, resulting in a constriction of self-knowledge and shallowness in the quality of relationships with others. The capacity to play with ideas in an imaginative way is lost. Instead, thinking takes on a concrete quality with a frightening equivalence between internal states and external reality (Fonagy & Target, 1996; Holmes, 2005).

The subsequent activation of state-dependent dissociated traumatic memories generates existential anxiety that oscillates between fear of engulfment and fear of abandonment (Renn, 2006, 2007), states of mind that may be expressed somatically (Krystal, 1988; McDougall, 1989; van der Kolk, 1989, 1994). These states, fantasies, and patterns of expectancies organise the person's subjective experience in everyday life. They emerge in the therapeutic relationship, being apparent in the patient's expressive behaviour and discourse style which, typically, is characterised by a sense of impending doom and catastrophe, as graphically described by Joseph (1989).

As a consequence of these vulnerabilities, the person's conscious coping strategies and fragile unconscious defensive structure may fragment in adulthood, particularly at moments of intense interpersonal stress when the self is felt to be endangered by loss of the primary attachment figure or love object. In such a context, the person's tenuous capacity for recognition and reflective functioning is compromised. There is a tendency to identify with the aggressor (Ferenczi, 1933; A. Freud, 1993) and wield power in a malign, coercive way in order to control the other and restore a sense of safety and security to the self. These dynamics become especially charged within therapeutic relationships, where authority, dependency, and desire intersect.

The activation and externalisation of dissociated self-states deriving from attachment trauma involving separation, loss, and abuse overwhelms the person's regulatory and reflective capacities. The ability to take the other's perspective is severely compromised when aspects of the current relationship align too closely with the original dissociated developmental trauma. Re-traumatisation of this kind, allied to a sense of shame, despair, powerlessness, and threat to the self, may culminate in extreme expressions of power and domination in the form of physical and sexual violence (Renn, 2003, 2006, 2007). In terms of Benjamin's theory, such a struggle for power reflects a breakdown in the intersubjective dimension of experience: the other is not recognised as a separate self with an equivalent centre of subjectivity but instead is related to predominantly as a toxic transferential object from the intrapsychic world (Benjamin, 1995).

These dynamics of power and recognition do not remain abstract; they come vividly alive in the therapeutic relationship, where authority, dependency, fear, and desire intersect. The next chapter turns to the moment-by-moment enactments through which these patterns are repeated, resisted, and potentially transformed within the analytic field.

References

Aron, L. (1996). *A meeting of minds: Mutuality in psychoanalysis*. Hillsdale, NJ: Analytic Press.

Aron, L. & Anderson, F. S. (eds). (1998). *Relational perspectives on the body*. Hillsdale, NJ: Analytic Press.

Bateman, A. & Fonagy, P. (2004). *Psychotherapy for borderline personality disorder: Mentalization-based treatment*. Oxford: Oxford University Press.

Beebe, B. & Lachmann, F. M. (1992). The contribution of mother-infant mutual influence to the origins of self- and object representations. In N. J. Skolnick & S. C. Warshaw (eds), *Relational perspectives in psychoanalysis* (pp. 83–117). Hillsdale, NJ: Analytic Press.

Beebe, B. & Lachmann, F. M. (2002). *Infant research and adult treatment: Co-constructing interactions*. Hillsdale, NJ: Analytic Press.

Benjamin, J. (1988). *The bonds of love: Psychoanalysis, feminism and the problem of domination*. New York: Pantheon.

Benjamin, J. (1992). Psychoanalysis as a vocation. *Psychoanalytic Dialogues*, 7(6), 781–802.

Benjamin, J. (1995). Recognition and destruction: An outline of intersubjectivity. In J. Benjamin, *Like subjects, love objects: Essays on recognition and sexual difference* (pp. 27–48). New Haven, CT: Yale University Press.

Bion, W. R. (1984). *Learning from experience*. London: Karnac Books.

Bollas, C. (1987). *The shadow of the object: Psychoanalysis of the unthought known*. London: Free Association Books.

Bowlby, J. (1997). *Attachment and loss, vol. 1. Attachment*. London: Pimlico.

Bowlby, J. (1998a). *Attachment and loss, vol. 2. Separation: Anxiety and Anger*. London: Pimlico.

Bowlby, J. (1998b). *Attachment and loss, vol. 3. Loss: Sadness and depression*. London: Pimlico.

Bromberg, P. M. (1998). *Standing in the spaces: essays on clinical process, trauma, and dissociation*. Hillsdale, NJ: Analytic Press.

Campbell, D. (1999). The role of the father in a pre-suicide state. In R. S. Perelberg (ed.), *Psychoanalytic understanding of violence and suicide* (pp. 75–86). London: Routledge.

Casement, P. (1990). *On learning from the patient*. London: Routledge.

Davies, J. M. & Frawley, M. G. (1994). *Treating the adult survivor of childhood sexual abuse*. New York: Basic Books.

Davies, J. M. (2004). Reply to commentaries. *Psychoanalytic Dialogues*, 14, 755–767.

de Zulueta, F. (1993). *From pain to violence: The traumatic roots of destructiveness*. London: Whurr Publishers.

Eng, D. L. & Han, S. (2001). A dialogue on racial melancholia. In S. Fairfield, L. Layton and C. Stack (eds), *Bringing the plague: Toward a postmodern psychoanalysis* (pp. 269–278). New York: Other Press.

Fairbairn, W. R. D. (1952). *Psychoanalytic studies of the personality*. London: Routledge.

Ferenczi, S. (1933). Confusion of tongues between adults and the child. In M. Balint (ed.), *Final contributions to the problems and methods of psycho-analysis* (pp. 156–167). London: Karnac Books.

Fletchman Smith, B. (2000). *Mental slavery: Psychoanalytic studies of Caribbean people*. London: Rebus Press.

Fonagy, P., Steele, M., Steele, H., Moran, G. S. & Higgitt, A. C. (1995). Attachment, the reflective self, and borderline states: The predictive specificity of the Adult Attachment Interview and pathological emotional development. In S. Goldberg, R. Muir & J. Kerr (eds), *Attachment theory: Social, developmental and clinical perspectives* (pp. 223–279). Hillsdale, NJ: Analytic Press.

Fonagy, P. (1999a). The transgenerational transmission of Holocaust trauma: Lessons learned from the analysis of an adolescent with obsessive-compulsive disorder. *Attachment & Human Development*, 1(1), 92–114.

Fonagy, P. (1999b). Towards understanding violence: The use of the body and the role of the father. In R. S. Perelberg (ed.), *Psychoanalytic understanding of violence and suicide* (pp. 53–72). London: Routledge.

Fonagy, P. & Target, M. (1996). Playing with reality: I. Theory of mind and the normal development of psychic reality. *International Journal of Psychoanalysis*, *77*, 217–233.

Fonagy, P. & Target, M. (2005). Bridging the transmission gap: An end to an important mystery of attachment research? *Attachment & Human Development*, 7(3), 333–343.

Fonagy, P., Steele, M., Steele, H., Moran, G. S. & Higgitt, A. C. (1995). The capacity for understanding mental states: The reflective self in parent and child and its significance for security of attachment. *Infant Mental Health Journal*, 12(3), 200–217.

Frankel, J. (2002). Exploring Ferenczi's concept of identification with the aggressor: Its role in trauma, everyday life, and the therapeutic relationship. *Psychoanalytic Dialogues*, 12, 101–139.

Frankel, J. (2006). Diagnosis-of-the-moment and what kind of good object the patient needs the analyst to be: Commentary on paper by Neil Skolnick. *Psychoanalytic Dialogues*, 16(1), 29–37.

Freud, A. (1993). *The ego and the mechanisms of defence*. London: Karnac Books.

Freud, S. (1905). Three essays on the theory of sexuality. In J. Strachey (ed.), *The standard edition of the complete psychological works of Sigmund Freud*, vol. 7 (pp. 125–245). London: Hogarth Press.

Freud, S. (1917). Mourning and melancholia. In J. Strachey (ed.), *The standard edition of the complete psychological works of Sigmund Freud*, vol. 14 (pp. 243–258). London: Hogarth Press.

Ghent, E. (1992). Process and paradox. *Psychoanalytic Dialogues*, 2(4), 135–160.

Grienenberger, J., Kelly, K. & Slade, A. (2005). Maternal reflective functioning, mother-infant affective communication, and infant attachment: Exploring the link between mental states and observed caregiving behaviour in the intergenerational transmission of attachment. *Attachment & Human Development*, 7(3), 299–311.

Hesse, E. & Main, M. (2000). Disorganized infant, child, and adult attachment: Collapse in behavioural and attentional strategies. *Journal of the American Psychoanalytic Association*, 48, 1097–1127.

Holmes, J. (1999). Ghosts in the consulting room: An attachment perspective on intergenerational transmission. *Attachment & Human Development*, 1(1), 115–131.

Holmes, J. (2005). Notes on mentalizing – old hat, or new wine? *British Journal of Psychotherapy*, 22(2), 179–197.

Joseph, B. (1989). Addiction to near-death. In M. Feldman & E. Bott Spillius (eds), *Psychic equilibrium and psychic change: Selected papers of Betty Joseph* (pp. 127–138). London: Karnac Books.

Khan, M. (1979). *Alienation in perversions*. London: Karnac Books.

Knox, J. (2001). Memories, fantasies, archetypes: An exploration of some connections between cognitive science and analytic science. *Journal of Analytical Psychology*, 46(4), 613–635.

Knox, J. (2003). *Archetype, attachment, analysis: Jungian psychology and the emergent mind*. Hove: Routledge.

Kraemer, S. B. (1996). Betwixt the dark and the daylight of maternal subjectivity: Meditations on the threshold. *Psychoanalytic Dialogues*, 6(6), 765–791.

Krystal, H. (1988). *Integration and self healing: Affect-trauma-alexithymia*. Hillsdale, NJ: Analytic Press.

Laing, R. D. & Esterson, A. (1964). *Sanity, madness and the family*. London: Tavistock.

Liotti, G. (1992). Disorganized/disoriented attachment in the etiology of the dissociative disorders. *Dissociation*, 5(4), 196–204.

Litowitz, B. E. (2002). Sexuality and textuality. *Journal of the American Psychoanalytic Association*, 50(1), 171–198.

Lyons-Ruth, K. (1991). Rapprochement or approchment: Mahler's theory reconsidered from the vantage point of recent research on early attachment relationships. *Psychoanalytic Psychology*, 8, 1–23.

Lyons-Ruth, K. & Jacobvitz, D. (1999). Attachment disorganization: Unresolved loss, relational violence and lapses in behavioural and attentional strategies. In J.

Cassidy & P. R. Shaver (eds), *Handbook of attachment: Theory, research and clinical applications* (pp. 520–554). New York: Guilford Press.

Mahler, M. S., Pine, F. & Bergman, A. (1985). *The psychological birth of the human infant: Symbiosis and individuation*. London: Karnac Books.

Main, M., Kaplan, N. & Cassidy, J. (1985). Security in infancy, childhood, and adulthood: A move to the level of representation. In I. Bretherton & E. Waters (eds), *Growing points of attachment theory and research* (pp. 66–104). Washington, DC: Society for Research in Child Development.

Mann, D. (1997). *Psychotherapy: An erotic relationship*. London: Routledge.

McDougall, J. (1989). *Theatres of the body: A psychoanalytic approach to psychosomatic illness*. London: Free Association Books.

McDougall, J. (1990). *Plea for a measure of insanity*. London: Free Association Books.

Milgram, S. (1974). *Obedience to authority*. London: Tavistock Publications.

Miller, A. (1991). Nicolae Ceausescu's vision of redemption. In *Breaking down the wall of silence* (pp. 97–113). London: Virago Press.

Mills, J. (2003). A phenomenology of becoming. In R. Frie (ed.), *Understanding experience: Psychotherapy and postmodernism* (pp. 116–136). London: Routledge.

Mitchell, S. A. (1993). *Hope and dread in psychoanalysis*. New York: Basic Books.

Mitchell, S. A. (1997). *Influence and autonomy in psychoanalysis*. Hillsdale, NJ: Analytic Press.

Mitchell, S. A. (2000). *Relationality: From attachment to intersubjectivity*. Hillsdale, NJ: Analytic Press.

Mitchell, S. A. & Black, M. J. (1996). *Freud and beyond: A history of modern psychoanalytic thought*. New York: Basic Books.

Orange, D. M. (1995). *Emotional understanding: Studies in psychoanalytic epistemology*. New York: Guilford Press.

Orbach, S. (1995). Countertransference and the false body. *Winnicott Studies*, 10.

Orbach, S. (1999). *The impossibility of sex*. Harmondsworth: Allen Lane.

Orbach, S. (2004). The John Bowlby Memorial Lecture 2003: The body in clinical practice. In K. White (ed.), *Touch: Attachment and the body*. London: Karnac Books.

Peck, C. J. (2003). Patterns of relating in the analytic field. *Psychoanalytic Inquiry*, 23 (2), 202–223.

Renn, P. (2003). The link between childhood trauma and later violent offending: The application of attachment theory in a probation setting. In F. Pfäfflin & G. Adshead (eds), *A matter of security: The application of attachment theory to forensic psychiatry and psychotherapy* (pp. 109–144). London: Jessica Kingsley Publishers.

Renn, P. (2006). Attachment, trauma and violence: Understanding destructiveness from an attachment theory perspective. In C. Harding (ed.), *Aggression and destructiveness: Psychoanalytic perspectives* (pp. 57–78). London: Routledge.

Renn, P. (2007). Stop thief! But what has been stolen and by whom? Discussion of paper by John Bowlby. *Attachment: New Directions in Psychotherapy and Relational Psychoanalysis*, 1 (1), 71–77.

Schacter, D. L. (1996). *Searching for memory: The brain, the mind, and the past*. New York: Basic Books.

Schore, A. (1991). Early superego development: The emergence of shame and narcissistic affect regulation in the practicing period. *Psychoanalysis and Contemporary Thought*, 14, 187–250.

Schore, A. (1994). *Affect regulation and the origin of the self: The neurobiology of emotional development*. Hillsdale, NJ: Lawrence Erlbaum Associates.

Schore, A. (2001). The effects of early relational trauma on right brain development, affect regulation and infant mental health. *Infant Mental Health Journal*, 22, 201–269.

Searles, H. (1993). The effort to drive the other person crazy: An element in the aetiology and psychotherapy of schizophrenia. In *Collected papers on schizophrenia and related subjects* (pp. 284–303). Madison, CT: International Universities Press.

Slade, A. (2005). Parental reflective functioning: An introduction. *Attachment & Human Development*, 7(3), 269–281.

Solomon, J., George, C. & De Jong, A. (1995). Children classified as controlling at age six: Evidence of disorganized representational strategies and aggression at home and at school. *Development and Psychopathology*, 7, 447–463.

Stern, D. N. (1985). *The interpersonal world of the infant: A view from psychoanalysis and developmental psychology*. New York: Basic Books.

Stoller, R. J. (1986). *Perversion: The erotic form of hatred*. London: Karnac Books.

Stubrin, J. P. (1994). *Sexualities and homosexualities* (trans. E. Reneboldi). London: Karnac Books.

Sullivan, H. S. (1953). *The interpersonal theory of psychiatry*. New York: W. W. Norton.

Sullivan, H. S. (1962). *Schizophrenia as a human process*. New York: W. W. Norton.

van der Kolk, B. A. (1989). The compulsion to repeat the trauma: Re-enactment, revictimization, and masochism. *Psychiatric Clinics of North America*, 2, 389–411.

van der Kolk, B. A. (1994). The body keeps the score: Memory and the evolving psychobiology of post-traumatic stress. *Harvard Review of Psychiatry*, 1, 253–265.

Winnicott, D. W. (1947). Hate in the counter-transference. *International Journal of Psycho-Analysis*, 30, 69–74.

Winnicott, D. W. (1958). The capacity to be alone. *International Journal of Psychoanalysis*, 39, 416–420.

Winnicott, D. W. (1960). Ego distortion in terms of true and false self. In D. W. Winnicott, *The maturational processes and the facilitating environment* (pp. 140–152). London: Hogarth Press.

Winnicott, D. W. (1967). Mirror-role of mother and family in child development. In D. W. Winnicott, *Playing and reality* (pp. 111–118). London: Tavistock Publications.

Winnicott, D. W. (1971). *Playing and reality*. London: Tavistock Publications.

Winnicott, D. W. (1974). Fear of breakdown. *International Review of Psycho-analysis*, 1, 103–107.

Part III

Relational Process and the Clinical Encounter

Introduction to Part III

Part I examined how relational patterns are formed and Part II explored how cumulative trauma shapes development and crosses generations. Part III turns to the consulting room to consider how these patterns emerge in therapeutic relationships and how transformation becomes possible.

The therapeutic relationship is not simply the context for clinical work, it is the primary site of procedural transformation. Patterns encoded in implicit memory and shaped by cumulative relational trauma do not present themselves solely as material to be interpreted. They are enacted in the quality of therapeutic engagement – in moments of connection and rupture, in transference and countertransference configurations, and in what can and cannot be spoken. The therapeutic relationship thus provides the conditions in which implicit relational patterns become available for recognition and revision, but it is within the patient's everyday relational life that these revisions acquire their fullest expression. Thus, transformation begins in the consulting room, but it is consolidated beyond it.

This section addresses some of the most challenging dimensions of relational clinical practice: recognising and working with enactments, navigating boundaries ethically, engaging sexual and erotic dimensions of transference, and extending relational thinking to severe presentations, including psychosis and states of intense anxiety.

The five chapters approach these issues from overlapping perspectives. Chapter 9 examines the therapeutic relationship as the vehicle for change. Drawing on research into implicit relational knowing, moments of meeting, and processes that extend beyond interpretation alone, it demonstrates how new procedural patterns emerge through sustained relational engagement characterised by attunement, rupture, and repair. Change is located in the micro-processes of interaction – in the therapist's capacity to recognise affective states, to remain present through enactments, and to restore connection after inevitable failures. The parallel with secure attachment is explicit: transformation depends not on perfection, but on reliable repair.

DOI: 10.4324/9781003789727-12

Chapter 10 focuses on enactments – those moments in which patient and therapist become caught in repetitive, often opaque relational patterns. Rather than treating enactments as failures or boundary breaches to be avoided, this chapter conceptualises them as inevitable expressions of implicit relational knowledge seeking recognition. Clinical work is reframed from preventing enactment to recognising, understanding, and working through it, with careful attention to ethical responsibility within co-created dynamics.

Chapter 11 builds on the clinical issues discussed in Chapter 10, with a focus on sexuality in the consulting room. Sexual feelings, erotic transference, and transference love are approached as central aspects of relational experience rather than marginal or merely problematic phenomena. This chapter explores how erotic dynamics can be held within a relational framework that honours their intensity and meaning while maintaining ethical containment, recognising sexuality as deeply intertwined with attachment, recognition, and power. Chapters 10 and 11 complement each other, providing a two-part exploration of the relational field. Chapter 10 establishes a relational framework for understanding enactments, boundaries, and self-disclosure, while Chapter 11 demonstrates these principles under conditions of maximum intensity in the sexual domain.

Chapter 12 extends relational thinking to work with psychotic and severe anxiety states. These presentations place exceptional demands on therapeutic capacity, requiring presence in the face of fragmentation, persecutory anxiety, and profound disconnection. Drawing on attachment and trauma perspectives, this chapter demonstrates how relational engagement – through provision of regulatory functions and recognition – remains possible and potentially transformative even in severe disturbance.

Chapter 13 turns outward. Having examined how relational patterns are recognised, enacted, and worked through in the consulting room, this chapter asks where transformation is ultimately realised. Drawing on Mitchell's sustained engagement with Connie's marriage, and on the author's commentary on Wachtel's account of relationality in everyday life, it argues that the patient's everyday relational world is not peripheral to analytic work but central to it. Procedural templates encoded in implicit memory are enacted most vividly and intensely in intimate relationships outside the consulting room. It is there, in the lived fabric of daily life, that new relational possibilities are most fully tested and consolidated. This chapter gives explicit form to a dimension that has remained implicit across the volume: that the consulting room is the space in which patterns are recognised and emotionally experienced, but everyday relationships are the arena in which they are transformed.

Together, these chapters establish that therapeutic change is procedural, occurring through lived experience rather than insight alone; that enactments are inevitable and clinically informative when recognised and worked through; that boundaries function to support relationship rather than constrain it; that sexual and erotic dimensions of transference require ethical engagement rather than avoidance; and that relational principles apply across the spectrum of clinical presentations, from neurotic conflict to severe pathology.

These insights have significant implications for clinical practice. If the therapeutic relationship is the primary medium of change, then clinical work requires sustained attention to the micro-processes of interaction – timing, affective tone, recognition and misrecognition – as well as to interpretation. Skill lies not in avoiding enactment, but in recognising and working within it, and in tolerating the uncertainty and vulnerability inherent in relational work.

Part III thus translates the developmental and theoretical frameworks established in Parts I and II into clinical practice. Understanding attachment, cumulative trauma, and intergenerational transmission is necessary but insufficient; clinicians must also know how to work with what emerges in the room. And what emerges is always relational: patterns seeking recognition, defences organised around safety, and longings shaped by prior experience.

The question animating this section is: how does change happen in practice? Not in theory, but in the lived reality of two people meeting over time, navigating connection and rupture, understanding and not-knowing. The answer proposed here is both simple and complex: change occurs through relationship – through being encountered, recognised, and allowed to become different within a sustained relationship.

9 The Therapeutic Relationship and the Process of Change

An Integrationist Perspective

Retrospective Reflection

This chapter was written at a point in my clinical and theoretical development when I was particularly concerned with understanding how change occurs within the therapeutic relationship, prior to interpretation or narrative elaboration. The emphasis on attachment theory, motivational systems, and neurobiological models reflects an attempt to articulate a framework capable of organising clinical attention to moment-to-moment process.

From the perspective of the present volume, some of this theoretical material overlaps with concepts developed elsewhere. Here, however, it is revisited not for exposition in its own right, but for its usefulness in illuminating how implicit relational patterns emerge and shift in vivo. The intention is not to rehearse theory, but to show how it quietly structures clinical perception: what is noticed, when intervention occurs, and how the therapist responds to subtle changes in affect, posture, and engagement.

The clinical work with Patricia remains central. Her difficulties in sustaining emotional contact, and the gradual emergence of vitality and agency within the therapeutic relationship, exemplify many of the processes explored throughout this book: cumulative relational trauma, impaired influence, procedural expectation, and the slow re-establishment of trust through attuned responsiveness. The brief illustration from John's history serves a complementary function, highlighting how dissociated affective states and deactivating attachment strategies may also shape the implicit relational field and require careful regulatory attunement. The theoretical frameworks invoked here are best understood as supporting this clinical process rather than explaining it away. The concept of cumulative relational trauma that informs this clinical material is developed theoretically in Chapter 5.

Revisiting this chapter now, I am struck by the continuity between its clinical concerns and the broader integrative stance developed later in the volume. While the language of theory has evolved, the underlying question remains the same: how therapeutic change becomes possible when experience is held, responded to, and gradually made available for reflection within a reliable relational context.

DOI: 10.4324/9781003789727-13

Introduction

The preceding chapters have established how early relational experience becomes encoded in implicit memory systems (Chapter 6) and transmitted across generations (Chapter 5). This chapter examines how such patterns emerge within the immediacy of the therapeutic relationship itself, often prior to interpretation or conscious reflection. Rather than locating change primarily in insight or narrative reconstruction, the focus here is on moment-to-moment relational process: how affect is regulated, how contact is sustained or disrupted, and how new experiences of influence and recognition gradually become possible.

The theoretical frameworks drawn upon in this chapter – attachment theory, motivational systems, and relational neuroscience – are introduced elsewhere in this volume. Here, they function less as objects of explanation than as orienting lenses that shape clinical attention. They inform what the therapist notices, how interventions are timed, and how shifts in engagement are understood as they unfold in vivo.

From this perspective, the therapeutic relationship itself becomes the primary site of change. Implicit relational expectations, shaped by earlier experience, are not simply represented or spoken about; they are enacted, tested, and potentially revised within the relational field of the session. The clinical material that follows illustrates how such processes emerge and how therapeutic responsiveness can support the gradual restoration of agency, vitality, and trust.

The work with Patricia provides the central clinical focus of the chapter. Her difficulties in sustaining emotional contact, and the slow emergence of greater aliveness within the therapeutic relationship, offer a concrete illustration of how procedural patterns shaped by earlier relational trauma may be transformed through sustained attunement and repair.

Attachment and Sexuality

Attachment theory may legitimately be criticised for omitting the importance of sexuality as a motivating factor in human behaviour. Attempts to rectify this omission have been made in recent years, most notably by Lichtenberg (2007, 2008) and Target (2007). Target (2007) found that mothers tended to ignore or avoid mirroring and marking their infants' affective state of sexual excitement. She argues that this unmentalised aspect of the child's attachment experience becomes split-off, forming part of an "alien self-structure". Such dissociated sexual dynamics may be enacted in subsequent attachment relationships and in the transference-countertransference matrix.

Although the mother-infant relationship is the focus of such research, my clinical experience strongly suggests that the father's influence on the developing child's sexuality is also highly significant and, therefore, likely to be enacted in the therapeutic relationship (Renn, 2013). Preliminary findings reported by Eagle (2007) and Lichtenberg (2007, 2008) support the ubiquitous influence of early attachment bonds on sexual relations in adulthood. Such findings provide compelling evidence that attachment strategies and implicitly encoded procedures formed in infancy influence, in a non-linear way, the playing out of the sexual system in adult romantic relationships (Mikulincer & Shaver, 2007).

From Liotti's perspective, relational disturbance may be understood in terms of conflict or disjunction between motivational systems, particularly where attachment needs coexist with expectations of danger or rejection. In such circumstances, proximity-seeking may simultaneously activate fear, leading to dissociation, freezing, or abrupt shifts in engagement. This framework is clinically useful not as a classificatory system, but as a way of understanding sudden changes in affect, posture, or relatedness within the session. In the work with Patricia, moments of withdrawal and disorganisation can be understood as reflecting such motivational conflict, becoming intelligible only when attended to as lived relational process rather than interpreted symbolically or retrospectively.

In clinical practice, then, attachment theory is used to conceptualise the developmental antecedents and interpersonal features of the patient's difficulties in living, particularly their implicitly encoded procedures for managing closeness and distance and separations and reunions in intimate relationships, and the influence of these phenomena on the formation of the therapeutic alliance (Lopez & Brennan, 2000).

Attachment theory and research provide both a particular way of listening to the patient's story and of understanding the clinical process (Slade, 1999). An aspect of this process involves identifying similarities in the complex dynamic interplay between the patient's early relational matrix and their current intimate relationships, including that with the therapist (Renn, 2003, 2006, 2008, 2012, 2013; Wachtel, 2008). This facilitates an understanding of the way in which archaic, nonconscious cognitive-affective mental models are being perpetuated in the here and now, actively mediating and distorting the person's attachment-related thoughts, feelings and behaviour, particularly at times of heightened emotional stress – how the silent relational past lives on in invisible ways in the interpersonal present (Renn, 2008b, 2012).

Attachment and Neuroscience

Contemporary neuroscience has provided a useful framework for understanding how early relational experience shapes affect regulation, stress responsivity, and the organisation of subjective experience. From an attachment perspective, repeated patterns of interaction between infant and caregiver contribute to the development of neural systems involved in arousal modulation, emotional processing, and relational expectancy. These systems are shaped not by isolated events, but by the cumulative quality of everyday relational exchanges.

Research on affect regulation has highlighted the role of right-hemisphere processes in the early organisation of emotional life. These non-verbal, affectively mediated forms of communication underpin the infant's emerging capacity to regulate internal states in relational contexts. Where caregiving is sufficiently attuned, regulatory capacities are gradually internalised; where attunement is inconsistent, frightening, or unavailable, the child may rely on dissociation or defensive withdrawal as adaptive strategies.

Within the therapeutic relationship, these early-established regulatory patterns often re-emerge implicitly rather than symbolically. The clinician's task is therefore not only interpretive, but regulatory: to provide a relational environment in which affect can be held, modulated, and gradually made available for reflection. Neuroscience, in this sense, does not offer a prescriptive technique, but supports a relational understanding of how therapeutic responsiveness can facilitate integration and change over time.

The Mirror Neuron System

The discovery of mirror processes has contributed to contemporary understandings of intersubjectivity by offering a neurobiological account of how emotional states may be shared at a pre-reflective level (Gallese, 2009; Rizzolatti et al., 2006). Rather than functioning as simple imitation, these processes support embodied resonance: one person registers aspects of another's experience through subtle shifts in posture, rhythm, tone, and expression.

Clinically, such resonance often precedes conscious formulation. The therapist may sense tension, withdrawal, or vitality in the body before these states are symbolised in language (Beebe et al., 2000; Stern, 1985, 2004). When held reflectively, this embodied knowing becomes part of the regulatory field, enabling affect to be recognised and gradually transformed. In this sense, mirror processes help illuminate how implicit relational experience becomes available for thought within an attuned therapeutic relationship.

Therapeutic Action

From a developmental perspective, therapeutic change involves shifts in implicit relational knowing – procedural patterns formed in early attachment relationships that continue to organise experience outside awareness (Lyons-Ruth et al., 1998; Stern, 2004). The Boston Change Process Study Group (2008, 2010) describe change as occurring through "now moments" and "moments of meeting", in which habitual expectations are briefly destabilised and new relational possibilities emerge.

Such moments are not primarily interpretive events. They arise within the implicit domain through coordinated affective engagement, often registered first in the body and only later articulated in words. When these encounters are recognised and integrated, implicit procedural models are modified, allowing experience to be reorganised at a more reflective level. In this sense, therapeutic action consists not only in narrative reconstruction but in the co-creation of new relational experience that gradually reshapes implicit expectations encoded through cumulative relational trauma.

In the therapeutic encounter, implicit modes of knowing are often first registered in the therapist's body before they reach symbolic form. Wallin's (2007) description of his work with "Ellen" offers a vivid illustration of how embodied attunement can become a gateway into the implicit relational field. His account also exemplifies how the therapist's mindful attention to bodily experience may open a "now moment" that shifts the intersubjective process.

Wallin writes of sitting with Ellen:

> I'm feeling calm, quietly taking in her presence without experiencing the familiar internal pressure to quickly respond. Staying with her, I'm also turning my attention to my breathing and my body. I have the not unfamiliar sense that I'm "knowing" her through my belly: my "gut sense" is that, as I'm relinquishing the lead, she's taking it.
>
> (Wallin, 2007, p. 321)

For me, Wallin's experience captures a form of body-based countertransference that is deeply consonant with contemporary neuroscience. The sense of "knowing through the belly" reflects the activation of the enteric nervous system – a vast neural network capable of registering affective states before they become symbolised. It also exemplifies what Gallese (2009) terms "embodied simulation": the therapist's body resonating with the patient's implicit emotional stance.

Mindful attention to these bodily shifts allows the therapist to participate consciously in the implicit domain, transforming background affect into shared experience. In this way, the therapist's embodied presence becomes part of the regulatory field, enabling a moment of meeting in which new relational possibilities can emerge.

Stern (2004) emphasises that anxiety on the part of the therapist may preclude engagement in "now moments", with the result that the opportunity for change at a key moment is lost. Whereas the BCPSG (2010) argue that change in the implicit domain may come about without the necessity of interpreting the experience in the explicit "verbal-reflective" domain, in line with Beebe and Lachmann (2002) they emphasise the interaction between the implicit, nonverbal domain and the explicit, verbal domain, arguing that exchanges on the verbal level are continually altering the dyad's timing, spatial organisation, affect, and arousal on a moment-to-moment basis in the implicit domain.

From this perspective, then, the process of change is conceptualised as the unfolding of an emergent intersubjective process characterised by the movement towards self-organisation in a context of destabilisation and perturbation. The model emphasises the fact that our experience is mediated by implicit, nonverbal representational models (Bowlby, 1988, 1998a; Fonagy & Target, 1997; Fonagy, 1999a; Shimmerlik, 2008). Therefore, accessing and making explicit invisible procedural ways of experiencing and relating – so that implicit memories can be subtly changed and encoded within second-order representational models – becomes a crucial aspect of therapeutic action (Fonagy et al., 2002).

These implicit procedural patterns often reveal themselves in the disjunction between a patient's conscious self-narrative and the dissociated affective states that organise behaviour. John's history offers a clear illustration of how unprocessed trauma and a deactivating attachment strategy can culminate in sudden, dysregulated enactments when mentalisation collapses (Renn, 2003).

John presented as a fundamentally passive, non-violent man who "wouldn't hurt a fly". Yet his relational history was marked by repeated episodes of intimate violence, typically occurring in the context of alcohol use and perceived rejection. This idealised self-representation functioned as a defensive structure that kept unbearable affect – shame, rage, fear of abandonment – out of awareness.

Under stress, however, these dissociated emotional states broke through. When confronted with relational threat, particularly the possibility of being left by his female partner, John's capacity to mentalise rapidly deteriorated. Alcohol served as a disinhibiting agent, loosening the fragile defensive scaffolding that ordinarily kept these affects at bay. In such moments, his unprocessed emotional turmoil, deriving from cumulative relational trauma, was enacted in the form of a violent rage. This was experienced by him as sudden and overwhelming, and as entirely alien to his conscious sense of self (Fonagy, 1999b).

Clinically, John's presentation highlights the central task of helping patients recognise and integrate dissociated affective states so that implicit relational patterns can be transformed rather than enacted. It also underscores the importance of the therapist's attuned presence in supporting the patient's capacity to remain within a window of tolerable affect, where mentalisation can be restored and new relational experience can emerge.

In this conceptual framework, pre-symbolic encounters in the implicit domain form the basis of intersubjective relatedness and promote the establishment of a secure-enough base from which to explore, express, and elaborate new forms of agency and shared experience (Lyons-Ruth et al., 1998; Stern et al., 1998b). In this sense, psychoanalysis may be seen as the active co-construction of a new way of experiencing self-with-other (Fonagy & Target, 1998; Fonagy, 1999a; Wachtel, 2008), and as identifying problematic patterns of organisation (Fosshage, 2011).

An Integrated Therapeutic Model

More generally, attachment theory and infant research demonstrate that psychological organisation is an adaptation aimed at preserving critical, life-sustaining relationships (Bowlby, 1988, 1998a; Lyons-Ruth & Block, 1996). As Slade (2004) points out, attachment classifications used for research purposes are simply ways of describing and organising implicitly encoded attachment phenomena. These silent phenomena, and the invisible processes and relational procedures they represent, are the focus of clinical work, not the classifications per se. A basic understanding of attachment theory and research sensitises the therapist to the nature and functioning of the attachment system and aids in the observation and recognition of attachment phenomena, as revealed in the patient's speech and behaviour (Slade, 2004; Main, 1991). The initial interview provides an ideal opportunity to begin to listen for attachment phenomena, as manifested in the patient's talk about their relationships with parents, partners and children (George, Kaplan & Main, 1985).

Clinical Illustration

The following case vignette of the first two sessions that I had with a new patient, "Patricia", illustrates the way in which the ideas emanating from attachment theory, narrative theory, mentalisation, affect regulation, neuroscience, implicit memory, and nonverbal communication can be applied to our clinical work, helping us to understand what is being subtly enacted in the therapeutic relationship (Renn, 2012, 2013; Fonagy et al., 2002; Stern, 2004). Whereas John's enactment emerged through collapse and disconnection, Patricia's transformation unfolded through restoration of contact and vitality.

Patricia, an attractive single woman in her early 30s, had self-referred. During the first session she spoke in considerable detail about her reasons for seeking therapy. She told a story of a fragmented family, losing contact with her father when she was six years old following her parents' separation and divorce. She had an unhappy school and home life, being bullied by a group of girls at school, and feeling excluded by the close alliance between her mother and older sister at home. She has an ongoing difficult relationship with her mother who, herself, was abandoned by her parents as a child and separated from her sister, whom she never saw again after being adopted (Renn, 2008a, 2008b).

Patricia had been diagnosed with depression in her early 20s, and was currently being treated with anti-depressants. She spoke of feeling emotionally dead and disconnected from herself and from others. Although in employment, everyday tasks were experienced as a huge burden weighing her down. She feared that her moods and behaviour were intractable and that change would not be possible because of an "imbalance in my brain chemistry". She had tried therapy once before, speaking in a dejected way of a failed, short-lived therapy with a female therapist some two years previously.

She described feeling angry, confused, and persecuted by the inconsiderate behaviour of family, friends, and work colleagues who, she believed, treated her in a dismissive and unfair way. She was plagued by guilt whenever she tried to assert herself, and so instead would ingratiate herself with others by putting their needs before her own, despite feeling a smouldering sense of injustice. All of this made matters worse as it left her feeling that she was over-controlling of herself and manipulative of others (Liotti, 1999; van der Kolk & Fisler, 1995).

A major reason for Patricia wanting therapy was a problem in sustaining intimate, sexual relationships with men. She said she felt like a child in relation to men, and that she allowed herself to be sexually used and emotionally abused by the men in her life. Despite this, she felt unable to leave the abusive relationships. More generally, Patricia spoke of feeling socially shy, inept and impulsive, physically ugly, morally prim, and sexually undesirable (Target, 2007; Lichtenberg, 2007, 2008).

Although I trust that I have set out Patricia's many and various difficulties in living in a relatively coherent way, her discourse style in telling me her story, as informed by research using the Adult Attachment Interview, was characterised by unfinished sentences, story lines that suddenly disappeared, only to merge with unrelated situations and expressions of hurt and injustice, and a pronounced difficulty in reflecting upon her experience in a collaborative way with me. There was an angry and excessive preoccupation with her past and present attachment relationships, with the boundaries between the two often seeming confused and diffuse (Hesse, 1999; Lyons-Ruth et al., 2005). I had considerable difficulty in getting a word in edgewise to bring her back to focus on a particular aspect of her life that she had started to tell me about, before she again wandered off at a tangent, starting a new thread and leaving the previous story unfinished and dangling in the air (Main, Kaplan & Cassidy, 1985).

Patricia seemed to be reliving in the here-and-now the emotional experiences that she was relating from the past, and to have little consciousness of me as a person to be connected with. Indeed, apart from gently guiding her back to the point of her story from time to time, I felt largely superfluous. However, I noted that whenever I shifted position in my chair, she would abruptly stop the flow of her monologue. This, I think, indicated that Patricia's attachment system was in a state of hyper-activation and that she was anxiously hyper-vigilant, monitoring my every move. Indeed, an informal benchmark for the establishment of a sense of safety and security with some patients is when they continue to speak during any movements that I might make. Moreover, a certain body-symmetry often develops, in that the patient's and my own shifts in position tend to mirror or mimic each other's. This may indicate the operation of the mirror neuron system and reflect the establishment of a bodily form of intersubjectivity.

I think it fair to assume that at a first meeting the patient is likely to feel somewhat vulnerable and to experience a degree of stress in the presence of a stranger, no matter how well-disguised this state might appear. This very stress tends to activate an archaic representational model and a discrete discourse style that communicates implicitly stored information to the therapist about the patient's current attachment expectations, early intersubjective experiences, and likely cumulative trauma. In this sense, the session does not merely reveal Patricia's difficulties; it reactivates the procedural residues of cumulative relational trauma within the therapeutic field itself. Although much of this could be discerned from the content of Patricia's story, the form of discourse in which she told it indicated a lack of "earned security" and an ongoing preoccupied state of mind in respect of attachment, together with a concomitant difficulty in managing her feelings and making sense of her own and other people's behaviour and mental states.

Preoccupied attachment is the adult corollary of infant ambivalent-resistant attachment organisation. It indicates an under-controlled emotion regulation system, as manifested by the hyper-activation of the attachment system, by an exaggerated style of emotion regulation, and by attempts to dramatically heighten emotional experience. The person's representational model tends to be characterised by dysregulated anger and an ever-present fear of rejection and abandonment. While there is conscious awareness of attachment affect, there is a cognitive disconnection between the affect and its cause and source. This creates confusion, anxiety, and a persistent sense of dread and foreboding.

Research indicates that this attachment state of mind develops in a relational matrix in which the preoccupied caregiver is inconsistently available and lacking contingent responsivity, or has an attachment need to keep the infant emotionally dependent on themselves. Thus, the caregiver focuses on negative affect to the exclusion of helping the child regulate their emotions. The failure to respond to attachment needs in ways that are consistent, contingent, and congruent with the infant's psychobiological states serves to keep the child intensely focused on the attachment relationship. This, in turn, reduces the chances of the child becoming emotionally independent of the caregiver.

In such infant-caregiver dyads the child is likely to develop an ambivalent-resistant pattern of attachment organisation that matches the caregiver's preoccupied state of mind, together with a style of regulating emotion that is preoccupied and under-regulated (Main et al., 1985; Peck, 2003). The initial indications were that Patricia's early attachment and intersubjective experiences had shaped and structured her inner world in these ways, as reflected in the attachment phenomena that I had observed and experienced at our first meeting (Slade, 1999).

Patricia began the second session in similar vein to the first, listing, in a rather hopeless and desultory way, the various problems she has in her relationships. Midway through the session she told me that she had gone out for a drink with work colleagues the previous evening. She described feeling sad and socially inept with her colleagues, hiding these feelings with a "smiley" exterior, and anxiously filling any gaps in the conversation with "empty words". In a rather heavy, defeated and despairing way, she said, "I expect I'll do the same here, so the therapy won't work".

Uncharacteristically, she left an interpersonal pause, and for the first time I felt invited to engage with her in a more direct way. I said in a quiet, soft voice: "But I might choose not to respond to your 'empty words' and leave a silence instead." Patricia looked at me sharply with an anxious, startled expression. I gazed back with bright eyes, smiled warmly, tilted my head to the left and, with a slightly quizzical, yet challenging, expression, raised my eyebrows and waited.

Patricia stared back, looking a bit panicky. I held her gaze and she started to laugh, shyly at first, covering her eyes with her left hand in embarrassment and peeping at me through her fingers. But she then seemed to surrender herself to the experience. Her laughter was prolonged and so delightful and infectious, that I found myself involuntarily joining in.

In between bouts of gurgling laughter she asked, "What have you done to me? I'm always the one that makes people laugh. No one ever makes me laugh. How did you do this? It's your training, isn't it?" Patricia went on to describe a "tingling feeling" in her throat, saying, "I know this therapy is going to work, I can feel it", adding, "I haven't felt so alive in years". However, she also said that her joy and pleasure were tinged with fear and trepidation, and that part of her wanted to flee from the room. In a playful tone of mock rebuke, and with bright smiling eyes, she said, "You're dangerous, you are!"

For someone like Patricia, who has been depressed for years and apparently habitually false and inauthentic in her relationships, to suddenly feel alive and emotionally connected must, indeed, have felt dangerous and alarming, the more so, perhaps, because of my gender. In terms of the BCPSG's model, Patricia and I shared a "now moment" that emerged in a rather sudden, dramatic and unpredictable way, catching us both by surprise and leading to a "moment of meeting" in the implicit/enactive domain. Initially, the mutual experience was predominantly body-based and nonverbal, and brought our implicit relational knowing into a changed state of "intersubjective consciousness".

From an attachment perspective, I would say that my implicit coordinated interactions with Patricia during the "now moment" experience were in the mid-range, that is, they were neither avoidant nor enmeshed but contingent and congruent to her state at that particular moment. Thus, there was also a degree of flexibility and variability which, given the way the interaction developed, seemed to have promoted a good enough sense of felt security in Patricia such that she could risk experiencing a relationship transformation in the here-and-now of the therapeutic encounter (Beebe et al., 2000).

The opportunity for this shared, intersubjective moment and new way of experiencing one another to emerge would, I think, have been lost had I chosen to interpret Patricia's expectation that the therapy would fail because of her "empty words". Could her very use of this phrase have implicitly influenced me to avoid using empty words of my own? No matter how clever and creative, an interpretation at that point would likely have deadened Patricia's lived experience and confirmed her expectation that spontaneous emotional connection is all but impossible for her.

I think this would also have been the case in the first session had I chosen to make a transference interpretation about her difficulty in leaving abusive relationships with men. Although I was not consciously aware of the implicit, nonverbal aspects of mutual influence occurring moment-to-moment in the first session (Beebe & Lachmann, 2002), I think that procedural/emotional aspects of the encounter paved the way for the "moment of meeting" to emerge in the second. This would seem to confirm Stern's (2004) contention that "making narratives involves not only words, but also direct experiences that are in the implicit domain" (p. 192). If John illustrates the collapse of mentalisation under stress, I would suggest that Patricia illustrates the possibility of its restoration through attuned engagement.

On a more general point, I often find with patients like Patricia, who carry a diagnosis of depression and who tend to self-pathologise in such a way, that they are not globally depressed. Rather, their depressed state appears to be context-dependent, in that it comes and goes, depending on the social situation they are in and the representational model or self-state that emerges in any given social context. The key factor here is emotional connectedness or intersubjective relatedness. Whenever the patient feels emotionally and authentically connected with another, the depression tends to lift, however temporarily. By contrast, feeling isolated and alone in the context of the ongoing absence of a companionable, intersubjective relationship is often accompanied by feelings of low mood and depression.

Helping the patient to recognise these shifts in mood, mental models, or self-states can, in itself, be therapeutic, bringing a sense of hope to counter despair. In this sense, the dramatic shift in Patricia's state of mind in the second session would suggest that the "now moment" experience constituted a transition from an archaic representational model to one that is actually available to her, but which needs to be strengthened and consolidated so that it becomes a more consistent aspect of her lived experience. My thinking in this regard accords with Wachtel's (2008) suggestion that paying attention to the patient's healthier, more adaptive ways of being, and examining the contextual nature of their moods and behaviour, "can greatly enhance our clinical work" (p. 73).

Conclusion

From the foregoing, it may be accepted that memory is important not as an account of history but as a means of communicating the nature of internal representations of self-other relationships. As we have seen, representational models are the invisible psychic structures that organise behaviour and experience in the present, mediating our expectations and predictions of self-other relationships deriving from the silent past (Bowlby, 1988, 1998b; Fonagy & Target, 1997; Fonagy & Target, 1998; Fonagy, 1999b; Fosshage, 2011; Renn, 2012; Stern, 2004; Wachtel, 2008). This being so, it is these structures themselves that need to be the focus of psychoanalytic work not the events that might have contributed to their development.

In the light of these findings, therapeutic work needs to focus on helping the patient to identify, and thus make visible, repetitive patterns of behaviour for which explicit memory can provide no explanation. Therefore, a key aspect of therapeutic action consists of the modification of implicit memories and the expression of dissociated emotions that motivate the procedures underpinning habitual ways of experiencing self with other (Fonagy & Target, 1998; Fonagy, 1999a; Renn, 2012; Wachtel, 2008). Many of these procedures may be highly dysfunctional but be based on powerful, yet outdated and largely nonconscious expectations generated by past experience of a cumulatively traumatic nature (Knox, 2003; Renn, 2003, 2006, 2008b; Wachtel, 2008; Wilkinson, 2010).

Given that such emotional procedures are not readily accessible for verbal report they may only become explicitly knowable when enacted in the implicit realm (Fonagy, 1999a; Lyons-Ruth, et al., 1998; Pally, 2005; Reis, 2009a, 2009b; Renn, 2012, 2013; Ringstrom, 2008; Shimmerlik, 2008; Stern et al., 1998b; Teicholz, 2009). From a clinical perspective, engaging focal attention and bringing the consciousness system to bear on implicit-procedural expectations and patterns of interaction is a vital therapeutic tool. Consciousness of previously nonconscious procedures, expectations, emotions and predictions facilitates choice, enhances behavioural and emotional regulation, and promotes therapeutic change (Fonagy & Target, 1998; Fonagy, 1999a; Fosshage, 2011; Pally, 2005; Schore, 1994; Renn, 2012; Shimmerlik, 2008; Wachtel, 2008).

In time, consciousness of the beliefs and expectations generated by emotional memories leads to changes in procedural rules and to the creation of second-order representational models of their inner experience (Eagle, 2003; Fonagy, 1999a; Sandler & Sandler, 1997). From a contemporary perspective, then, psychoanalysis works by modifying procedural mental models and the accompanying emotions that are generated and enacted in particular self-other relationships (Bowlby, 1988). Therefore, bringing implicit-procedural structures into conscious focus in an emotionally meaningful way is a critical component of therapeutic action (Eagle, 2003; Fonagy, 1999a; Fosshage, 2011; Orange, 1995; Pally, 2005; Renn, 2012, 2013;

Schore, 1994, 2001; Sandler & Sandler, 1997; Shimmerlik, 2008; Stern et al., 1998a; Wachtel, 2008).

Given the implicit and explicit dimensions of therapeutic action, it is, of course, important that therapists become aware of the implicit-procedural aspects of their own affect and behaviour, as well as that of the patient. This facilitates implicit/enactive aspects of the exchange being brought into the verbal/reflective domain. This dual aspect of therapeutic action suggests that the therapist functions both to enact and to reflect on the interaction (Fosshage, 2011; Pally, 2005; Reis, 2009a, 2009b; Renn, 2012; Wallin, 2007). From a neuroscience perspective, utilising the explicit, declarative system of the hippocampus allows optimal implicit-procedural interactions between patient and therapist to become more strongly encoded in the patient's amygdala and basal ganglia of the implicit memory system with the outcome that these more optimal procedures are activated automatically and habitually (Pally, 2005). The clinical challenges and opportunities presented by such enactments, including questions of boundary and responsibility, are examined directly in Chapter 10.

As previously noted, this process links the nonverbal and verbal representational domains of the brain, thereby facilitating the transfer of implicit-procedural information in the right hemisphere to explicit or declarative systems in the left. Thus, body-based, visceral-somatic experience is symbolically transformed into emotional and intentional states of mind that become available for reflection and regulation (Damasio, 2000; Schore, 1994). From an attachment theory perspective, these new forms of agency and shared experiences become encoded in the systems of implicit-procedural memory as second-order representational models (Fonagy, 1999a).

Taken together, the clinical material in this chapter illustrates how therapeutic action unfolds through the transformation of implicit relational procedures rather than through interpretation alone. Whether the attachment system is hyperactivated, as in Patricia's case, or defensively deactivated, as in John's, the therapist's task is to participate in and regulate the implicit relational field so that dissociated or unintegrated states can be safely experienced, recognised, and gradually symbolised. In this sense, therapeutic change emerges not from insight imposed from above, but from the co-creation of new relational experience – moments in which previously unthinkable affect becomes thinkable, and previously foreclosed forms of agency and connection begin to take shape.

The processes described here – implicit relational knowing, moments of meeting, procedural transformation – constitute the foundation of therapeutic action. Yet such moments inevitably give rise to complexity: erotic dynamics that challenge boundaries, and work with severe disturbance that requires particular responsiveness. These respective challenges are addressed in Chapters 11 and 12. First, Chapter 10 explores enactments and boundary dilemmas directly, viewing them not as deviations but as opportunities to bring about therapeutic change by engaging with implicit relational processes that such relational dynamics represent.

References

Beebe, B., Jaffe, J., Lachmann, F. M., Feldstein, S., Crown, C. & Jasnow, M. (2000). Systems models in development and psychoanalysis: The case of vocal rhythm coordination and attachment. *Infant Mental Health Journal*, 21, 99–122.

Beebe, B. & Lachmann, F. M. (2002). *Infant research and adult treatment: Co-constructing interactions*. Hillsdale, NJ: Analytic Press.

Beebe, B., Knoblauch, S., Rustin, J. & Sorter, D. (2005). *Forms of intersubjectivity in infant research and adult treatment: A systems view*. New York: Other Press.

Boston Change Process Study Group. (2008). Forms of relational meaning: Issues in the relations between the implicit and reflective–verbal domains. *Psychoanalytic Dialogues*, 18(2), 125–148.

Boston Change Process Study Group. (2010). *Change in psychotherapy: A unifying paradigm*. New York: Norton.

Bowlby, J. (1988). *A secure base: Clinical applications of attachment theory*. London: Routledge.

Bowlby, J. (1998a). *Attachment and loss, vol. 2. Separation: Anxiety and anger*. London: Pimlico.

Bowlby, J. (1998b). *Attachment and loss, vol. 3. Loss, sadness and depression*. London: Penguin.

Bruschweiler-Stern, N., Harrison, A. M., Lyons-Ruth, K., Morgan, A. C., Nahum, J. P., Sander, L. W., Stern, D. N. & Tronick, E. Z. (2007). The foundational level of psychodynamic meaning: Implicit process in relation to conflict, defence and the dynamic unconscious. *International Journal of Psychoanalysis*, 88, 843–860.

Damasio, A. (2000). *The feeling of what happens: Body, emotion and the making of consciousness*. London: Vintage.

Eagle, M. N. (2003). Clinical implications of attachment theory. *Psychoanalytic Inquiry*, 23, 27–53.

Eagle, M. (2007). Attachment and sexuality. In D. Diamond, S. J. Blatt & J. D. Lichtenberg (eds), *Attachment and sexuality* (pp. 27–50). New York: Analytic Press.

Fonagy, P. (1999a). Memory and therapeutic action. *International Journal of Psycho-Analysis*, 80, 215–223.

Fonagy, P. (1999b). The transgenerational transmission of holocaust trauma: Lessons learned from the analysis of an adolescent with obsessive-compulsive disorder. *Attachment & Human Development*, 1(1), 92–114.

Fonagy, P. & Target, M. (1997). Perspectives on the recovered memory debate. In J. Sandler & P. Fonagy (eds), *Recovered memories of abuse: True or false?* pp. 183–216. London: Karnac Books.

Fonagy, P. & Target, M. (1998). An interpersonal view of the infant. In A. Hurry (ed.), *Psychoanalysis and developmental therapy* (pp. 3–31). London: Karnac Books.

Fonagy, P., Gergely, G., Jurist, E. L. & Target, M. (2002). *Affect regulation, mentalisation, and the development of the self*. New York: Other Press.

Fosshage, J. L. (2011). How do we "know" what we "know?" And change what we "know?" *Psychoanalytic Dialogues*, 21, 55–74.

Gallese, V. (2009). Mirror neurons, embodied simulation, and the neural basis of social identification. *Psychoanalytic Dialogues*, 19, 519–536.

George, C., Kaplan, N. & Main, M. (1985). Adult attachment interview. APA PsycTests. doi:10.1037/t02879-000.

Hesse, E. (1999). The Adult Attachment Interview: Historical and current perspectives. In J. Cassidy & P. R. Shaver (eds), *Handbook of attachment: Theory, research and clinical applications* (pp. 395–433). New York: Guilford Press.

Knox, J. (2003). *Archetype, attachment, analysis: Jungian psychology and the emergent mind*. Hove: Routledge.

Lichtenberg, J. D. (2007). A discussion of eight essays that propel attachment and sexual theories into the 21st century. In D. Diamond, S. J. Blatt & J. D. Lichtenberg (eds), *Attachment and sexuality* (pp. 237–261). New York: Analytic Press.

Lichtenberg, J. D. (2008) *Sensuality and sexuality across the divide of shame*. New York: Analytic Press.

Liotti, G. (1999). Understanding the dissociative processes: The contribution of attachment theory. *Psychoanalytic Inquiry*, 19(5), 757–783.

Lopez, F. G. & Brennan, K. A. (2000). Dynamic processes underlying adult attachment organisation. *Journal of Counseling Psychology*, 47(3), 283–300.

Lyons-Ruth, K. & Block, D. (1996). The disturbed caregiving system: Relations among childhood trauma, maternal caregiving, and infant affect and attachment. *Infant Mental Health Journal*, 17(3), 257–275.

Lyons-Ruth, K., Bronfman, E. & Atwood, G. (1999). A relational diathesis model of hostile–helpless states of mind. In J. Solomon & C. George (eds), *Attachment disorganisation* (pp. 33–70). New York: Guilford Press.

Lyons-Ruth, K., Bruschweiler-Stern, N., Harrison, A. M., Morgan, A. C., Nahum, J. P., Sander, L. W., Stern, D. N. & Tronick, E. Z. (1998). Implicit relational knowing: Its role in development and psychoanalytic treatment. *Infant Mental Health Journal*, 19(3), 282–289.

Lyons-Ruth, K., Yellin, C., Melnick, S. & Atwood, G. (2005). Expanding the concept of unresolved mental states. *Development and Psychopathology*, 17, 1–23.

Main, M. (1991). Metacognitive knowledge, metacognitive monitoring, and coherent vs. incoherent models of attachment. In C. M. Parkes, J. Stevenson-Hinde & P. Marris (eds), *Attachment across the life cycle* (pp. 127–159). Hove: Routledge.

Main, M., Kaplan, N. & Cassidy, J. (1985). Security in infancy, childhood, and adulthood: A move to the level of representation. *Monographs of the Society for Research in Child Development*, 50(1–2), 66–104.

Mikulincer, M. and Shaver, P.R. (2007). A behavioural systems perspective on the psychodynamics of attachment and sexuality. In D. Diamond, S. J. Blatt & J. D. Lichtenberg (eds), *Attachment and sexuality* (pp. 51–78). New York: Analytic Press.

Orange, D. M. (1995). *Emotional understanding: Studies in psychoanalytic epistemology*. New York: Guilford Press.

Pally, R. (2005). A neuroscience perspective on forms of intersubjectivity. In B. Beebe, S. Knoblauch, J. Rustin & D. Sorter (eds), *Forms of intersubjectivity in infant research and adult treatment* (pp. 191–241). New York: Other Press.

Peck, S. D. (2003). Measuring sensitivity moment-by-moment. *Attachment & Human Development*, 5(1), 38–63.

Reis, B. (2009a). Performative and enactive features of psychoanalytic witnessing. *International Journal of Psychoanalysis*, 90, 1359–1372.

Reis, B. (2009b). We: Commentary on papers by Trevarthen, Ammaniti & Trentini & Gallese. *Psychoanalytic Dialogues*, 19, 565–579.

Renn, P. (2003). The link between childhood trauma and later violent offending: The application of attachment theory in a probation setting. In F. Pfäfflin & G. Adshead (eds), *A matter of security: The application of attachment theory to forensic psychiatry and psychotherapy* (pp. 109–144). London: Jessica Kingsley.

Renn, P. (2006). Attachment, trauma and violence: understanding destructiveness from an attachment theory perspective. In C. Harding (ed.), *Aggression and destructiveness: Psychoanalytic perspectives* (pp. 57–78). Hove: Routledge.

Renn, P. (2008a). Attachment, Affect Regulation and Trauma: The Transmission of Patterns Across Generations. In E. Arnold & B. Hawkes (eds), *Internalising the historical past: Issues for separation and moving on* (pp. 24–33). Newcastle: Cambridge Scholars Press.

Renn, P. (2008b). The relational past as lived in the interpersonal present: Using attachment theory to understand early trauma and later troubled relationships. In E. Arnold & B. Hawkes (eds), *Internalising the historical past: Issues for separation and moving on* (pp. 59–69). Newcastle: Cambridge Scholars Press.

Renn, P. (2012). *The silent past and the invisible present: Memory, trauma, and representation in psychotherapy*. New York: Routledge.

Renn, P. (2013). Moments of Meeting: The Relational Challenges of Sexuality in the Consulting Room. *British Journal of Psychotherapy*, 29(2), 135–153.

Ringstrom, P. A. (2008). Improvisation and mutual inductive identification in couples therapy. *Psychoanalytic Dialogues*, 18, 390–402.

Rizzolatti, G., Fogassi, L. & Gallese, V. (2006). Mirrors in the mind. *Scientific American*, November (pp. 54–69).

Sandler, J. & Sandler, A.-M. (1997). A psychoanalytic theory of repression and the unconscious. In J. Sandler & P. Fonagy (eds), *Recovered memories of abuse* (pp. 163–181). London: Karnac Books.

Schore, A. N. (1994). *Affect regulation and the origin of the self*. Hillsdale, NJ: Lawrence Erlbaum.

Schore, A. N. (2001). The effects of early relational trauma on right brain development. *Infant Mental Health Journal*, 22, 201–269.

Shimmerlik, S. M. (2008). The implicit domain in couples and couple therapy. *Psychoanalytic Dialogues*, 18, 371–389.

Slade, A. (1999). Attachment theory and research. In J. Cassidy & P. R. Shaver (eds), *Handbook of attachment* (pp. 575–594). New York: Guilford Press.

Slade, A. (2004). The move from categories to process. *Infant Mental Health Journal*, 25(4), 269–283.

Stern, D. N. (1985). *The interpersonal world of the infant*. New York: Basic Books.

Stern, D. N. (2004). *The present moment in psychotherapy and everyday life*. New York: Norton.

Stern, D. N., Sander, L. W., Nahum, J. P., Harrison, A. M., Lyons-Ruth, K., Morgan, A. C., Bruschweiler-Stern, N. & Tronick, E. Z. (1998a). The process of therapeutic change involving implicit knowledge. *Infant Mental Health Journal*, 19(3), 300–308.

Stern, D. N., Sander, L. W., Nahum, J. P., Harrison, A. M., Lyons-Ruth, K., Morgan, A. C., Bruschweiler-Stern, N. & Tronick, E. Z. (1998b). Non-interpretive mechanisms in psychoanalytic therapy: The "something more" then interpretation. *International Journal of Psychoanalysis*, 79, 903–921.

Target, M. (2007). Sexuality and attachment. *Psychoanalytic Inquiry*, 27, 448–464.

Teicholz, J. G. (2009). Introduction to "optimal responsiveness and the therapist's reaction to the patient's unresponsiveness". *Psychoanalytic Psychology*, 26(3), 235–238.

van der Kolk, B. A. & Fisler, R. (1995). Dissociation and the fragmentary nature of traumatic memories: Overview and exploratory study. *Journal of Traumatic Stress, 8*(4), 505–521.

Wachtel, P. L. (2008). *Relational theory and the practice of psychotherapy*. New York: Guilford Press.

Wallin, D. J. (2007). *Attachment in psychotherapy*. New York: Guilford Press.

Wilkinson, M. (2010). *Changing minds in therapy: Emotion, attachment, trauma and neurobiology*. New York: Norton.

10 A Relational Perspective on Enactments, Boundary Violations, and Self Disclosure

Retrospective Reflection

This chapter was written during a period in which my clinical thinking was increasingly shaped by relational psychoanalysis and by the recognition that enactments are not exceptional failures of technique but ubiquitous features of therapeutic work. At the time, much of the literature on enactment was concerned with questions of responsibility, boundary management, and ethical risk, often framed in polarised terms of permissiveness versus restraint. Returning to this material now, I am struck by how enactments can be more usefully understood as sites where unmentalised experience and cumulative relational trauma come alive within the therapeutic relationship.

From the perspective developed across this volume, enactments may be seen as expressions of implicit relational knowledge shaped by early attachment disturbance, dissociation, and repeated failures of recognition. They emerge not because therapists or patients have erred, but because certain forms of experience cannot yet be thought or symbolised. In this sense, enactments represent both danger and opportunity: danger when they remain unrecognised or defensively managed, and opportunity when they can be reflected upon, contained, and worked through relationally. The developmental and intergenerational origins of such cumulative relational trauma are examined in detail in Chapter 5.

This chapter therefore occupies a pivotal position in the book. It builds on earlier discussions of implicit process and cumulative trauma, while preparing the ground for later chapters on sexuality, violence, and severe disturbance. Read retrospectively, it reflects a growing appreciation of the ethical responsibility involved in relational work, alongside a commitment to understanding enactments not as technical failures but as potential pathways toward recognition, repair, and developmental change. These dynamics become even more charged when sexuality enters the relational field, a theme taken up directly in the following chapter.

DOI: 10.4324/9781003789727-14

Introduction

This chapter extends the developmental and relational foundations established earlier in the volume by examining enactments as lived expressions of implicit relational process. Whereas previous chapters explored the formation of dissociated self-states, cumulative trauma, and the neurobiological underpinnings of affect regulation, the focus here shifts to how these histories become active within the therapeutic relationship itself. Enactments, boundary dilemmas, and self-disclosure are approached not as technical deviations but as inevitable moments in which unrepresented experience presses for recognition. In this sense, the chapter serves as a conceptual hinge, linking the developmental material that precedes it with the later discussions of sexuality, violence, and severe disturbance. The memory systems through which such implicit processes are encoded and maintained are discussed in Chapter 6. Chapter 11 extends this discussion into the domain of sexuality, where implicit relational processes often manifest with particular intensity.

Jacobs (1986) was one of the first to use the term *enactment* in an analytic context. He conceptualised enactment as a subtle interlocking of the transference and countertransference that operates outside of conscious awareness, often through nonverbal means. More recently, he suggests that the root of enactments lies in mutually regulating and self-regulating behaviours (Jacobs, 2005). Enactments may also be understood in terms of Sandler's (1976) theory of role-responsiveness.

Elaborating on Sandler's theory, Gabbard (1996) contends that countertransference enactments represent a joint creation that involves contributions from both the therapist and the patient. Whereas the patient may actualise an internal scenario within the therapeutic relationship, resulting in the therapist playing a role scripted by the patient's internal world, the dimensions of the role enacted by the therapist will be coloured by their own subjectivity. This reflects the fact that therapists bring their own wishes, needs, and desires to the therapeutic situation, as well as their own traumatic histories.

A Relational Perspective

On discussing countertransference enactments, Mitchell (1993) compares a relational/intersubjective model to that employed by Freud (1905e) in his brief analysis of Dora. Mitchell (1993) argues that Freud's focus on intrapsychic neurotic conflict invalidated Dora's subjective experience of trauma and abuse, and perpetuated, in the countertransference, her victimisation by the men in her life. Thus, Mitchell (1997) cautions us to guard against enacting or re-enacting in the transference/countertransference matrix aspects of the patient's original traumatic experience or abusive relationships by blaming, victimising or, indeed, seducing the patient. Seductive behaviour by the therapist may include a countertransferential wish to rescue or parent the patient, thereby encouraging a regressive dependency

(Herman, 1992; Blum, 1994). Mitchell (1997) emphasises that awareness of countertransference tendencies of these kinds requires continual self-reflective responsiveness to the material being presented.

Although we may well heed Mitchell's (1997) cautionary words about being drawn into enactments with our patients, as doing so is likely to interfere with the development of a good working relationship, Davies and Frawley (1994) argue that traumatic transference/countertransference enactments are inevitable. Evolving out of their work with adult survivors of childhood sexual abuse, the authors delineate eight positions, as expressed within four relational matrices. In a similar way to Sandler's (1976) theory of role-responsiveness, these positions, roles, or self-states may alternately be enacted by the therapist and patient in the transference/countertransference matrix. They include the uninvolved, non-abusing parent and the neglected child, the sadistic abuser and the helpless, impotently enraged victim, the idealised, omnipotent rescuer and the entitled child who demands to be rescued, and the seducer and the seduced. Davies and Frawley (1994) suggest that mutually dissociated traumatic experience is particularly susceptible to being enacted in the intensity of the therapeutic relationship.

A Trauma Perspective

This view is endorsed by Herman (1992). Writing from a traumatology perspective, she describes the traumatic or vicarious countertransference, suggesting that the patient's dissociated trauma may overwhelm the therapist. One among several reactions to this situation is the therapist's need to defend against unbearable feelings of helplessness. Thus, therapists who ordinarily are scrupulous in observing the limits of the therapeutic frame may find themselves violating the bounds of the therapy relationship and assuming the role of rescuer, thereby disempowering the patient. Under the intense pressures of the traumatic transference/countertransference, the therapist may take on an advocacy role for the patient, feel obliged to extend the limits of therapy sessions, allow frequent emergency contacts between sessions, and answer phone calls late at night or when on vacation. Herman (1992) points out that the therapist's defence against feelings of helplessness may lead to a stance of grandiose special-ness or omnipotence, with the attendant risk of extreme boundary violations, up to and including sexual intimacy. Such violations are frequently rationalised on the basis of the patient's desperate need for rescue and the therapist's extraordinary gifts as a rescuer.

Non-abusive Enactments

Paradoxically, as the relational literature shows, non-abusive enactments may lead to profound therapeutic change (Stern, 2010), enhancing a sense of felt security and the capacities for affect regulation and mentalisation (Fonagy, 2008). Indeed, there is broad agreement that countertransference enactments are not only ubiquitous but also potentially useful (Aron, 1990; Chused, 1991; Renik, 1993; Renn, 2012). A relational perspective, informed by developmental studies, holds that the adequate repair of non-abusive ruptures constitutes therapeutic action, with the consequent gain of a constructive outcome (Beebe & Lachmann, 1994, 2002; Benjamin, 1995; Fonagy, 1998; Roth & Fonagy, 1996). Similarly, Chused (1991) argues that the benefit for the therapy is not the enactment itself, but rather the eventual understanding that derives from the enactment.

Crucially, then, the outcome depends on how the enactment is worked with in the therapeutic relationship – can it be contained and collaboratively explored, validating the patient's subjective reality and thereby provide a shared, co-constructed emotional experience as the rupture to the working alliance is repaired? Or will it replicate past abusive relationships and thus risk re-traumatising the patient? In this context, Gabbard (1996) strikes a note of caution, stating: "Integral to the notion that countertransference enactments are useful is the understanding that analysts must catch themselves in the midst of the enactment when it is manifesting itself in an *attenuated* or *partial form*" (pp. 84–85, italics in original). This need for timely recognition becomes especially crucial when enactments take an erotic form, as explored in the next chapter.

Enactments and Self-Disclosure

Mitchell (1988) argues that in order to work relationally the therapist must be prepared to take risks in the service of connecting with the patient in a real and authentic way. Thus, passionate feelings of love and hate may often arise between the analyst and patient. In this context, Mitchell (2000) observes that relationally oriented clinicians are often "portrayed as wild analysts, doing and saying anything that occurs to them in an unrestrained fashion" (p. 127). He believes that this criticism is "ill-founded", arguing that relational analysts approach their clinical work with caution and responsibility (p. 127). However, Mitchell (1997) does make it quite clear that the question for the contemporary relational therapist is not *whether* to share countertransferential thoughts and feelings but rather *when and to what extent*. In his view, selective disclosure of the countertransference may function to help the patient and therapist connect on an emotional level and thereby open up, vitalise, and validate their subjective experience, providing them with a sense of being valued and understood. Handled insensitively, however, disclosure may close down and deaden the patient's experience.

Clearly, then, the decision to disclose requires a responsible, sensitive, and judicious approach by the therapist that takes full account of the need to protect the patient's personal integrity and boundaries. As Mitchell (1997) puts it, a delicate balance needs to be achieved whereby the therapist is neither excessively emotionally detached from the patient nor excessively intimate and intrusive.

Maroda (2010) defines self-disclosure as "any verbal expression of personal feelings or information on the therapist's part, whether deliberate or not" (p. 108). Self-evidently, self-disclosure can have a positive or a negative impact on the therapeutic relationship. Indeed, Aron (1990) advocates allowing the patient access to the therapist's subjectivity, in terms of disclosing their thoughts, feelings and fantasies. He argues that this leads to an acknowledgement by the patient of the therapist as a separate subject. This notwithstanding, in order to protect the patient, we need to ask ourselves what the therapeutic purpose is of self-disclosure, whether it would be useful, digressive, or disruptive, and what the motivation is for disclosing personal feelings or information.

Moreover, as Wachtel (2008) observes, considerations about how much, when, and how to disclose require sophisticated, reflective, and patient-centred attention. In broad terms, the therapeutic benefits accruing from sensitive and responsible self-disclosure are that it may confirm the patient's sense of reality, break impasses and repair ruptures, promote new relational experiences, and facilitate shared states of mind and emotional honesty.

Although it is generally agreed that self-disclosure works best when there is a strong therapeutic alliance, both Maroda (2010) and Wachtel (2008) emphasise that we cannot always correctly appraise when disclosure will be helpful and growth-promoting, and that we must, therefore, be prepared to work with the consequences of getting it wrong. These authors also stress that the interactions with the patient need to be individualised, recognising that what is appropriate for one patient may well not be so for another. As Maroda (2010) puts it, "therapeutic self-disclosure is a result of intuitive and artistic responses in a unique, creative moment with an individual client" (p. 113). As ever, the context needs to be taken into account in deciding whether or not to self-disclose. As Mitchell (2000) notes: "Love and hate in long-term relationships, like the analytic relationship, do not just happen. They are shaped and cultivated within contexts that are constructed slowly, over time" (p. 129).

Erotic Transference/Countertransference Issues

With regard to erotic feelings in the therapeutic dyad, Mann (1997) argues that the therapist's open recognition of their erotic desire and subjectivity indicates a mature awareness of the differentiation between self and other which may help to preclude the sexual abuse of the patient. Indeed, Celenza (2010) argues that erotic excitement is a normal and expectable experience in the therapeutic encounter. Moreover, she suggests that "all treatments must revolve, at some level, around the question 'Why can't we be lovers?'" (p. 66). In order to avoid boundary violations, she contends that this question "must be reckoned with and will involve the use of erotic arousal in the dyad" (p. 66).

Indeed, Searles (1965) argues that successful work depends on the therapist recognising and reciprocating the patient's transference love without acting on these feelings. Mann (1997), however, advises against the disclosure of erotic feelings to the patient, a view generally shared by Maroda (2010), who states: "I am really against disclosure of erotic countertransference, with rare exceptions" (p. 218). For his part, Mitchell states:

> Ultimately it falls to the analyst to make decisions about the constructive versus destructive implications of various affects in both participants in the analytic process, even though there is no way to make those judgments purely objectively. Part of the analyst's responsibility is to participate in and enjoy that love, while it seems facilitative of the analytic process, but not to enjoy that love so much that it becomes a vehicle for the analyst's own pleasure in a way that occludes his focus on the patient's well-being.
>
> (Mitchell, 2000, p. 139)

Chapter 11 takes up these questions in detail, examining how erotic transference and countertransference test the therapist's capacity for reflection, containment, and ethical responsibility.

Indeed, Gabbard (1996) notes that the powerful and compelling nature of sexual and loving feelings may override the therapist's reflectiveness. Countertransference enactments of such feelings occur along a continuum from overt sexual relations between patient and therapist at one end, to subtle forms of enactment involving partial transference gratifications of a verbal and nonverbal nature within the boundaries of the therapeutic frame at the other end. He states that:

> In any countertransference enactment, analysts must strive to determine the relative balance of their own contributions versus the patient's contributions. A key part of that reflective process is determining which role, if any, one is playing in the patient's internal cast of characters.
>
> (Gabbard, 1996, p. 86)

Mutual Influence

Therapy, then, is an inherently intense, intimate, and risky business. Trauma, like madness, may be contagious, that is, be transmitted interpersonally. Mutual or bi-directional influence, on both a conscious and unconscious level of mental functioning, is continuously in operation, for good or for ill. Therapist and patient get drawn into inevitable transference/countertransference enactments on a continuum of seriousness under the sway of nonconscious representational models, unresolved trauma, and mutual dissociation. Enactments can be a force for therapeutic change or a vehicle for abuse and re-traumatisation (Renn, 2012, 2013). This dichotomy is succinctly summed up by Kernberg (1995) who, in discussing the erotic aspects of the transference/countertransference, notes: "There is probably no other area of psychoanalytic treatment in which the potentials for acting out and for growth experiences are so intimately condensed" (p. 114).

The Therapeutic Frame

Clearly, then, safeguards are required. The therapeutic frame includes an adherence to ethical codes and guidelines designed to protect the patient from abuse and boundary violations. These may be reinforced by regular supervision and membership of a peer support group. Maintaining the frame in a consistent and ethically boundaried way may allow the patient to feel sufficiently safe and free to develop, explore, and express erotic and aggressive feelings in relation to the therapist, thereby providing grist to the therapeutic mill.

The frame, then, provides a containing structure and creates the conditions for attachment security and the symbolic elaboration of dissociated and unmentalised wishes, desires, and affects deriving from unresolved trauma, loss, neglect, or abuse. Conversely, breaching the frame by, for example, adopting a position of omnipotent rescuer may unwittingly disempower the patient and foreclose on opportunities for therapeutic change.

Conclusion

Enactments are not aberrations or technical lapses but intrinsic features of relational work, arising at the points where dissociation, cumulative trauma, and unformulated experience strain the capacity for reflection. They signal moments in which the therapeutic relationship is asked to bear what has previously been unthinkable. The task is not to prevent enactment but to recognise it, survive it, and gradually transform it into shared meaning.

Such work requires a disciplined balance of openness and containment, emotional honesty, and ethical responsibility. When therapists can acknowledge and reflect upon their participation in enactments, these moments become opportunities for repair through which new relational expectations take shape. In this way, enactments illuminate the developmental principles that underpin change throughout the volume: the co-construction of safety, the restoration of reflective functioning, and the emergence of new patterns of relating. The next chapter applies these principles to the relational challenges of sexuality, where enactments often become most vivid and clinically consequential.

This chapter stands at a pivotal point in the book. It links the developmental and trauma-based formulations of earlier chapters with the more complex material that follows, including erotic transference, boundary dilemmas, and severe disturbance. Across these contexts, the evidence remains consistent: it is the interactive, emotion-regulating dimension of the therapeutic relationship – the capacity to engage, withstand, and repair – that drives intrapsychic change and supports the patient's movement towards greater integration (Gabbard & Hobday, 2012; Roth & Fonagy, 1996; Schore, 1994; Stern et al., 1998; Shedler, 2010).

Taken together, the themes explored here – enactment, self-disclosure, erotic transference, mutual influence, and the therapeutic frame – prepare the ground for the chapters that follow. The clinical challenges of sexuality, aggression, and severe disturbance cannot be understood without appreciating how dissociated experience becomes enacted in the relational field, nor can they be worked with without a secure frame capable of containing such intensity. The next chapters build directly on this relational sensibility, showing how the same principles of recognition, regulation, and repair apply when the stakes are highest and the material most charged. In certain domains – particularly sexuality – these enactments may become especially fraught, exposing both the risks and possibilities inherent in relational work. These principles are taken forward in Chapter 11 in relation to sexuality and erotic transference, and in Chapter 12 in work with severe disturbance.

References

Aron, L. (1990). One-person and two-person psychologies and the method of psychoanalysis. *Psychoanalytic Psychology*, 7, 475–485.

Beebe, B. & Lachmann, F. M. (1994). Representation and internalisation in infancy: Three principles of saliency. *Psychoanalytic Psychology*, 11, 127–165.

Benjamin, J. (1995). Recognition and destruction: An outline of intersubjectivity. In *Like subjects, love objects: Essays on recognition and sexual difference* (pp. 27–48). New Haven, CT: Yale University Press.

Blum, H. P. (1994). *Reconstruction in psychoanalysis: Childhood revisited and recreated*. Madison, CT: International Universities Press.

Celenza, A. (2010). The analyst's need and desire. *Psychoanalytic Dialogues*, 20, 60–69.

Chused, J. F. (1991). The evocative power of enactments. *Journal of the American Psychoanalytic Association*, 39, 615–639.

Davies, J. M. & Frawley, M. G. (1994). *Treating the adult survivor of childhood sexual abuse*. New York: Basic Books.

Fonagy, P. (1998). Moments of change in psychoanalytic theory: Discussion of a new theory of psychic change. *Infant Mental Health Journal*, 19(3), 346–353.

Fonagy, P. (2008). The mentalization-focused approach to social development. In F. N. Busch (Ed.), *Mentalization: Theoretical considerations, research findings, and clinical implications* (pp. 3–56). New York: Analytic Press.

Freud, S. (1905e). Fragment of an analysis of a case of hysteria (Dora). In J. Strachey (ed.), *The standard edition of the complete psychological works of Sigmund Freud*, vol. 7 (pp. 1–122). London: Hogarth Press.

Gabbard, G. O. (1996). *Love and hate in the analytic setting*. Northvale, NJ: Jason Aronson.

Gabbard, G. O. & Hobday, G. S. (2012). A psychoanalytic perspective on ethics, self-deception and the corrupt physician. *British Journal of Psychotherapy*, 28(2), 235–248.

Herman, J. L. (1992). *Trauma and recovery*. New York: Basic Books.

Jacobs, T. J. (1986). On countertransference enactments. *Journal of the American Psychoanalytic Association*, 34, 289–307.

Jacobs, T. J. (2005). Discussion of forms of intersubjectivity in infant research and adult treatment. In B. Beebe, S. Knoblauch, J. Rustin & D. Sorter (eds), *Forms of intersubjectivity in infant research and adult treatment: A systems view* (pp. 165–189). New York: Other Press.

Kernberg, O. F. (1995). *Love relations: Normality and pathology*. New Haven, CT: Yale University Press.

Mann, D. (1997). *Psychotherapy: An erotic relationship*. London: Routledge.

Maroda, K. J. (2010). *Psychodynamic techniques: Working with emotion in the therapeutic relationship*. New York: Guilford Press.

Mitchell, S. A. (1988). *Relational concepts in psychoanalysis: An integration*. Cambridge, MA: Harvard University Press.

Mitchell, S. A. (1993). *Hope and dread in psychoanalysis*. New York: Basic Books.

Mitchell, S. A. (1997). *Influence and autonomy in psychoanalysis*. Hillsdale, NJ: Analytic Press.

Mitchell, S. A. (2000). *Relationality: From attachment to intersubjectivity*. Hillsdale, NJ: Analytic Press.

Renik, O. (1993). Analytic interaction: Conceptualising technique in light of the analyst's irreducible subjectivity. *Psychoanalytic Quarterly*, 62, 553–571.

Renn, P. (2012). *The silent past and the invisible present: Memory, trauma, and representation in psychotherapy*. New York: Routledge.

Renn, P. (2013). Moments of Meeting: The relational challenges of sexuality in the consulting room. *British Journal of Psychotherapy*, 29(2), 135–153.

Roth, A. and Fonagy, P. (1996). *What works for whom? A critical review of psychotherapy research*. New York: Guilford Press.

Sandler, J. (1976). Countertransference and role-responsiveness. *International Review of Psychoanalysis*, 3, 43–47.

Schore, A. N. (1994). *Affect regulation and the origin of the self: The neurobiology of emotional development*. Hillsdale, NJ: Lawrence Erlbaum Associates.

Searles, H. F. (1965). Oedipal love in the countertransference. In H. F. Searles, *Collected papers on schizophrenia and related subjects*. Madison, CT: International Universities Press.

Shedler, J. (2010). The efficacy of psychodynamic psychotherapy. *American Psychologist*, 65 (2), 98–109.

Stern, D. B. (2010). *Partners in thought: Working with unformulated experience, dissociation, and enactment*. New York: Routledge.

Stern, D. N., Sander, L. W., Nahum, J. P., Harrison, A. M., Lyons-Ruth, K., Morgan, A. C., Bruschweiler-Stern, N. and Tronick, E. Z. (1998). The process of therapeutic change involving implicit knowledge: Some implications of developmental observations for adult psychotherapy. *Infant Mental Health Journal*, 19 (3), 300–308.

Wachtel, P. L. (2008). *Relational theory and the practice of psychotherapy*. New York: Guilford Press.

11 Moments of Meeting

The Relational Challenges of Sexuality in the Consulting Room

Retrospective Reflection

This chapter addresses sexuality not as a discrete clinical topic, but as a domain in which the relational dynamics explored throughout this volume become unusually concentrated and visible. Sexual feelings in the consulting room often bring implicit expectations, vulnerabilities, and long-established patterns of influence into sharp relief, exposing both patient and therapist to heightened affect and ethical complexity.

Written at a time when relational approaches were increasingly foregrounding authenticity and mutual influence, the chapter reflects my concern to think carefully about how such ideas can be held without collapsing the therapeutic frame or disavowing asymmetries of power. Sexuality, perhaps more than any other aspect of clinical work, tests the clinician's capacity to remain present, reflective, and contained while tolerating uncertainty and emotional intensity.

From the perspective developed later in this volume, the clinical material can be understood as illustrating the impact of cumulative relational trauma as it emerges in the therapeutic relationship. The patient's sexualised communications function not simply as expressions of desire, but as attempts to establish influence, secure recognition, and manage fears of loss and abandonment. The therapeutic task, therefore, lies less in managing content than in attending to process: how meanings are co-created, how enactments are perceived, and how repair becomes possible without foreclosure or retreat. The concept of cumulative relational trauma that informs this understanding is developed theoretically and developmentally in Chapter 5.

Revisiting this chapter now, I am struck by the extent to which the clinical dilemmas it explores remain current. While theoretical language has evolved, the ethical and relational challenges posed by sexuality in the consulting room have not diminished. If anything, they underscore the necessity of a clinical stance that is neither avoidant nor permissive, but grounded in sustained reflection, relational responsibility, and a commitment to keeping experience thinkable. In this sense, the chapter builds directly on the relational and developmental foundations established in Chapter 10.

DOI: 10.4324/9781003789727-15

Introduction

In recent years, a number of commentators have noted a dearth of articles discussing sexuality in psychoanalysis. It is argued that this reflects a paradigm shift from Freud's drive theory, which views sexuality and aggression as innate constitutional forces motivating mental functioning and human behaviour, to post-Freudian developmental theories that emphasise preoedipal conflict and the regulation of affects in the mother-infant relationship (Budd, 2001; Green, 1996; Harding, 2001; Holmes, 2007; Litowitz, 2002; Mann, 1997; Stein, 1998; Target, 2007; Tyson, 2002). The new paradigm is apparent in the respective theorising of Fairbairn, Winnicott, Balint, and Bowlby from an object relations/attachment perspective. Here, mental functioning is seen as motivated by, and organised around, relational needs rather than centred on instinctual wishes and innate drives of sexuality and aggression. These authors have, in turn, influenced the development of relational psychoanalysis in the USA.

Contemporary practitioners have shifted attention from an exclusive focus on the patient's unconscious process to include the complex relational context within which personal subjectivity develops. Mitchell (1988) argues that in order to work relationally the therapist must be prepared to take risks in the service of connecting with the patient in a real, humane and authentic way. In this context, Ogden (2004) observes that the quality of intimacy developed between therapist and patient will include feelings of camaraderie, playfulness, compassion, healthy flirtatiousness, charm, and enlivening humour. In contrast, a classical approach, at least as defined by Friedman (2010), views any emotional reaction or responsiveness by the analyst as a countertransference enactment that would be detrimental to the treatment. I would suggest that such polarised views have become increasingly redundant and outdated and thus risk parodying theoretical and technical differences between relational and traditional approaches within contemporary psychoanalysis.

That said, Harding (2001) and Target (2007) argue that the transference-countertransference relationship has come to be influenced by the new relational paradigm with the unintended consequence that the transference has become de-sexualised. While writers such as Budd (2001) and Mann (1997) view this shift as retrograde, resulting in the de-eroticisation of the therapeutic relationship and the concomitant disappearance of sexuality from psychoanalysis, others, either explicitly or implicitly, suggest that relational and developmental perspectives are misunderstood in this respect and have much to contribute to understanding and working with sexuality in clinical practice (Fonagy, 2008a; Gabbard, 1996; Lichtenberg, 2007, 2008; Litowitz, 2002; Target, 2007; Tyson, 2002).

This chapter builds upon the general relational and developmental framework for understanding enactments developed in Chapter 10, focusing specifically on sexuality as a domain in which these dynamics become intensified and ethically charged. I illustrate theoretical points with a clinical case study, a development of previously published work (Renn, 2012).

Sexuality, Attachment, and Dissociation

Contemporary developmental perspectives emphasise that sexual excitation is present from infancy and that affect regulation strategies are co-created during repeated attachment transactions. When early attachment contexts are characterised by dramatic abuse or cumulative relational trauma, the capacity to mentalise is compromised, and unmentalised sexual experience may become located within a dissociated part of the self (Fonagy et al., 2002; Schore, 1994).

Research by Target (2007) found that mothers have particular difficulty in mirroring and marking their infants' sexual excitement. Instead of responding in an attuned, contingent way, mothers often ignored or avoided the child's affective state of sexual arousal. In consequence, this unmentalised aspect of the child's attachment experience may become split-off or dissociated, forming part of an "alien self" which is implicitly encoded in representational models of self-other relationships. Such dissociated sexual dynamics may be enacted in subsequent attachment relationships and in the transference-countertransference matrix. Target (2007) concludes that the pressure of sexuality, in the context of an alien self-structure, pushes for externalisation and thus may be manifested in the transgression of personal boundaries.

Writing from an attachment and trauma perspective, Liotti (1999) argues that in order to avoid the painful, confusing experience of dissociation to which a contradictory, multiple self-representation developed in childhood is linked, the person may defensively inhibit the attachment system by choosing, consciously or unconsciously, to activate a competing motivational system, such as the sexual system. According to Liotti (1999), the activation of the sexual system creates "the basis for promiscuity and for the construction of any significant relationships according to the roles of seducer and the seduced" (p. 771). He argues that the choice of the sexual system is facilitated if the person has been sexually abused by an attachment figure, being selected in the service of avoiding painful attachment experiences associated with loss, rejection, and abandonment.

The Relational Challenges of Sexuality in the Consulting Room

While we may agree that there has, indeed, been a hiatus in recent decades in the discussion of psychosexuality in psychoanalysis, more recent publications and research findings show that sexuality is, in fact, very much alive, if not exactly well, in the consulting room. In light of such research, and the contemporary relational focus on intersubjectivity and co-construction, it is no longer feasible to speak only of the patient's sexual feelings for the therapist in isolation from the therapist's erotic desire for the patient (Gabbard, 1996; Lichtenberg, 2008; Mann, 1997).

Indeed, Rodgers (2011) found that sexual attraction by or for a patient is recognised as widespread and prevalent among therapists. Her review of the literature shows that up to 90% of therapists report having been sexually attracted to at least one patient. Similarly, Martin et al. (2011) found that sexuality is a common aspect of the therapeutic relationship. However, both Rodgers (2011) and Martin et al. (2011) found that therapists were anxious and confused about how to work ethically with sexual attraction and the erotic transference, and that there is a need for a clearer understanding of what constitutes a therapeutic, as opposed to a non-therapeutic, response to sexuality in the consulting room. Their respective findings highlight a gap in training about patient-therapist sexual attraction and the erotic transference/countertransference, as well as a lack in the literature addressing the potential benefits of working ethically with such clinical issues.

In this context, it is posited that the retreat from an analytic focus on sexuality occurred in parallel to a fundamental change in the role of the therapist from that of an objective neutral observer who is free from the patient's direct influence in a classical one-person psychology to that of an active participant in a more intimate two-person relational process in which mutual influence is an inherent and ubiquitous aspect of the intersubjective field (Aron, 1996; Benjamin, 1995; Gabbard, 1996; Target, 2007). That said, contemporary psychoanalytic thinking acknowledges that the analytic process incorporates both a two-person and a one-person psychology, and thus is both intrapsychic and interpersonal (Benjamin, 1992; Gabbard, 1996).

Given this, both parties bring their habitual patterns of relating and loving to the therapeutic work. From a contemporary perspective, then, the countertransference is viewed as a joint creation involving mutual influence and bi-directional contributions from both patient and therapist (Aron, 1996). Thus, the erotic transference is shaped by ongoing mutual enactments between the dyad, reflecting their respective self and object experiences (Gabbard, 1996). However, Gabbard (1996) argues that there is considerable gender fluidity in the roles played by both therapist and patient, suggesting that a variety of transferences may emerge that involve both homosexual and heterosexual longings and desires. Rodgers (2011), though, notes "the infrequency with which homoerotic countertransference is discussed, even by gay authors" (p. 267).

Self-Disclosure and Erotic Countertransference

Accepting that the therapeutic relationship is increasingly characterised by openness, emotional intimacy, and mutual enactments, it is perhaps not surprising that therapists are less comfortable exploring sexual material with their patients for fear of crossing a sexual or ethical boundary. With regard to sexualised self-disclosure, the intensity of an eroticised relationship may result in the "as if" nature of the transference/countertransference being lost by both therapist and patient, with the reflective, analysing function of the therapist becoming overwhelmed (Gabbard, 1996).

Lichtenberg (2008) posits that one or other of a number of different forms of love may emerge in the therapeutic relationship: attachment love, romantic love, lustful love, love without lust, and transference love. With regard to lustful love, Gabbard (1996) and Gabbard and Hobday (2012) emphasise that it is the therapist's reflective, analysing role that differentiates love and sexual desire in the analytic situation from love in everyday life. This notwithstanding, contemporary psychoanalysis holds that the patient's love is both real, in terms of a unique current relationship, and unreal, in that it has elements of past internalised object relations that are reactivated in the therapeutic dyad.

Power, Asymmetry, and Ethical Responsibility

Celenza and Gabbard (2007) found that where sexual boundary violations have occurred, they are the endpoint of a gradual shift in the therapeutic frame characterised by the therapist attempting to maintain a positive relationship with the patient by avoiding conflict or hostility, often through inappropriate self-disclosure. This, in turn, may reflect the therapist's desperate desire to be idealised, loved, and sexually desired by the patient (Gabbard, 1996). Moreover, Gabbard and Hobday (2012) observe that when therapists cross sexual boundaries they typically engage in self-deceptive practices whereby they rationalise their boundary-violating behaviour. Such practices include: minimising the adverse impact of sexualising the therapeutic relationship on the patient, overstating the psychological health of the patient, rationalising the boundary violation as patient initiated, experiencing a sense of being in love with a soul mate, and claiming that such practice is acceptable in their therapeutic community.

Sexual boundary violations, by their very nature, reflect an abuse of power whereby the patient's vulnerability and need for care is exploited (Gabbard & Hobday, 2012). Given this, Celenza (2010) argues that the power differential is a necessary tool of the therapeutic relationship and that therapists need to be mindful of power in all its complexity rather than defensively denying its existence. Such denial may result in a mutual enactment whereby the therapist's attraction to the patient and the patient's desire for the therapist's love, merge to create "a powerful addictive cycle of erotic excitement" (Celenza & Gabbard, 2007, p. 179).

In Gabbard and Hobday's (2012) study, a number of therapists justified their boundary violations by arguing that the practice was acceptable within their particular theoretical orientation and community. In contrast to such a view, which clearly places the patient at risk, I suggest that an overly anxious response to sexuality in the consulting room reflects a similarly defensive stance which may have the effect of foreclosing recognition of the patient's desire and experience.

More generally, Feltham (2007) questions whether this might slide into a defensive mind-set of "take no risks". He suggests that the therapist who plays everything by the book, employing a set of rigid prescriptions to maintain an ethical frame, may foreclose the space to develop a humane, intersubjective relationship, leaving the patient with a sense of having been abused by a too rigidly correct therapist. The "take no risks" approach may, therefore, end up breaching the "do no harm" injunction – in effect, the treatment becomes iatrogenic, that is, actively harmful.

Aron (1996) argues that a significant factor influencing therapists to adopt such an overly rigid style of working is anxiety about becoming known by their patients. Indeed, he suggests that one reason why therapists "choose" the analytic profession is because we have conflicts over intimacy, not least sexual intimacy. In Winnicottian terms (Winnicott, 1965), it may be said that we have a desire to be found and known by the other and a defensive need to remain hidden and "incommunicado". Such anxiety, particularly with regard to sexuality, may preclude the therapist from adopting a more spontaneous, intersubjective style of working that characterises a relational/developmental perspective, and which may be said to reflect the basic difference in approach between traditional and relational practice. Though, again, I think that such differences are often overstated.

Case Illustration

In chapter 7 of my book *The Silent Past and the Invisible Present* (Renn, 2012), I illustrate the way in which I used a contemporary relational model, informed by a developmental sensitivity, to engage with a patient, "Katarina", who had expressed a desire to have a sexual relationship with me. I subsequently presented a brief extract from this clinical vignette, together with a number of additional clinical observations, in the *British Journal of Psychotherapy* (Renn, 2013), which I reproduce here. I would see the vignette as an example of *one* way of working with the relational challenges of sexuality as they emerge within a unique intersubjective relationship. The clinical material that follows illustrates how the enactment processes described in Chapter 10 become intensified when sexuality enters the therapeutic relationship.

Before presenting the case, I should emphasise that Katarina has given permission for an account of our work together to be published. Her name has been changed and personal circumstances disguised in order to protect her identity.

Katarina is a 38-year-old married woman with an eight-year-old son whom I have been seeing twice a week for five years, working face-to-face. A recurrent theme in the therapy has been Katarina's ambivalence about becoming too closely attached to me because of fearing that she will lose me in some way – that I will die, get ill, change profession, or retire. She also fears that she is "too much" for me and that I find the sessions with her "boring". Thus, becoming attached is experienced as dangerous because of an implicit expectation that it will lead to abandonment and loss. Such fears are repeatedly expressed in Katarina's narrative, which is characterised by the anticipation of catastrophic losses and betrayals. Paradoxically, but perhaps in an attempt to counter such fears of loss and abandonment, Katarina has attempted to extend the boundaries of the therapy, questioning, almost from the outset, why it is not possible for us to have a personal relationship. Thus, she has repeatedly expressed a wish to meet for coffee or lunch, saying that seeing me twice a week under the constraints of therapy "isn't enough".

From the details that emerged about Katarina's formative experiences growing up in Eastern Europe, her anxiety about becoming attached, and concomitant expectation of loss, have a basis in reality, in terms of insecure attachment to both parents, cumulative developmental trauma, and the intergenerational transmission of fearful parental states of mind. Meaningful emotional communication in her family of origin was stilted and inhibited, and has remained so in the intervening years. Her previous therapist died unexpectedly shortly after Katarina left her country of origin to settle in the UK. Although there is no reported history of childhood sexual abuse, Katarina has engaged in sexual sadomasochism with strangers in the past.

The following encounter occurred some two years into the therapy. Katarina began by saying that coming to see me feels like "cheating" on her husband because she enjoys talking to me so much and can do so in ways that she can't with him. She went on to say again how disappointed and frustrated she feels in not being able to have a relationship with me outside of the sessions; that she would like to meet with me for lunch, and that she has been wondering what it would be like to have sex with me. At the weekend Katarina had visited a historic town in the north of England with her husband and son. Although this had been a pleasurable excursion, she had felt disconnected from her husband and child and had started to think about how much more enjoyable it would have been if she had been there with me. After relating these thoughts and desires, she fell silent and looked forlornly out of the window in a rather trance-like, dissociated way.

This was the first time that Katarina had spoken openly about sex in relation to me, and I felt in something of a dilemma as to how to respond without leaving her feeling rejected and invalidated. Indeed, this moment exemplifies what Chapter 10 described as the "danger and opportunity" inherent in enactments: danger of re-traumatisation through rejection or rigidity, opportunity for transformation through attuned recognition.

Whereas in the past I have dealt with her bids to have a personal relationship by emphasising that this would destroy the therapeutic relationship, together with any benefit that she might be gaining from it, on this occasion, albeit without much pre-reflective thought, I chose to respond in a different way. I said that I, too, might feel disappointed and frustrated that we can't meet for a coffee or lunch; that I, too, might have wondered what it would be like to have sex with her; that had we met under different circumstances, I, too, might have wanted to develop an intimate friendship with her. With a smile and twinkle in my eye, I ended by saying "although I'm old enough to be your father, the thought of spending a romantic weekend with you in York sounds very appealing. It's such a damned shame I'm your therapist, isn't it?"

Katarina turned to look at me, smiling and laughing with me as we shared the transgressive idea of a naughty weekend away together. After this, there was a perceptible shift in her state of mind – from a familiar state of disappointment, deprivation, and frustration to a more reflective state in which she could engage with me in exploring the various difficulties in living with which she is currently struggling.

Taken out of context, my response to Katarina may be viewed as egregious or, at the very least, controversial, particularly by an analyst such as Friedman (2010), who, as noted above, argues that any emotional response to a patient constitutes acting out in the countertransference. Even when the context is taken into account, I would agree with Mitchell's (2000) contention that "All analytic writing necessarily lends itself to misreading in one direction or another" (p. 126). This is particularly likely to be the case when discussing a somewhat taboo subject, such as sexual attraction between therapist and patient, and the contentious issue of self-disclosure. Moreover, despite the prevalence of such phenomena, as discussed above, the paucity of papers on the specific topic of sexual attraction may reflect what Britton (1997) refers to as "publication anxiety". He suggests that a common source of such anxiety is "fear of recrimination by affiliated colleagues and possible exile from them" (p. 14). In this overall context, I must confess to harbouring a degree of "publication anxiety" myself.

What, then, prompted my somewhat risky, improvisatory (Ringstrom, 2008) interaction with Katarina, with its playful and flirtatious "might have beens" and "if onlys"? And what led me to conclude that it would be safe to do so, and that Katarina would hear my self-disclosure in the way that it was intended? Perhaps more to the point, why did I think that my particular response to her bid for an intimate relationship would be useful and therapeutically beneficial to her at this particular moment, when I have responded in a more formal, pragmatic way to such bids on past occasions?

First and foremost, I recall feeling immensely touched that Katarina had shared such intimate thoughts and feelings with me, leaving herself exquisitely vulnerable to a humiliating rebuff. I knew that what I said in response had to touch her in return in a way that created a meaningful emotional connection between us in the real relationship – that my response had to be real and heartfelt, rather than defensive or judgmental. This reflects Mitchell's (1997) contention that selective self-disclosure may function to help the patient and therapist connect on an emotional level and, thereby, open up, vitalize and validate the patient's subjective experience, providing them with a sense of being valued and understood. As Mitchell (1997) puts it, a delicate balance needs to be achieved whereby the therapist is neither excessively emotionally detached from the patient nor excessively intimate and intrusive.

Indeed, in response to Gabbard and Lester's (1995) argument that self-disclosure of the countertransference constitutes a "slippery slope" that will inevitably result in disastrous sexual transgressions with patients, Mitchell (1997) contends that "there is also a slippery slope from excessive analytic restraint and avoidance of countertransference to a frozen, disastrous detachment from the patient" (p. 198). He asserts that "Excessive emotional detachment is just as fertile ground for sexual violations as excessive intimacy" (p. 198). That said, and in case there should be any doubt in the mind of the reader, I should emphasise that Mitchell is absolutely clear that relational psychoanalysis proscribes any form of sexual relations with patients.

From a relational perspective, then, what I actually ended up saying was an attempt to find a balance between affirming Katarina as a woman with desires, on the one hand, and maintaining the boundaries of the therapeutic frame, on the other hand. Given the context that I set out above, and the establishment of a strong therapeutic alliance, I suspected that she knew that I knew that we were relating in the "as if" or pretend mode (Fonagy et al., 2002), and that this, in itself, made it safe to play with such highly charged material. This is not to deny that the stakes were high and that there could have been dire consequences had I got it wrong. Indeed, Gabbard and Hobday (2012) emphasise that the therapist's problems with mentalisation are central to discrepancies between what the therapist intended and its actual impact on the patient. Casement (1990) argues that the empathic recognition and understanding of the patient's perspective is enhanced by developing the capacities of "internal supervision" and "trial identification" (p. 34). Following the Boston Change Process Study Group (2010), I would suggest that much of this reflective process is occurring non-consciously in the implicit domain of being and relating (see discussion below).

As to my immediate motivation in responding as I did, my main conscious concern was to avoid hurting or humiliating Katarina, but also to relate to her with emotional honesty and promote a new relational experience. Had I stayed silent, or proffered a cogent but emotionally distancing interpretation, this would have replicated the constricted pattern of communication in her family of origin. In this sense, responding in such a way would, itself, have constituted an enactment, and, I suspect, have left Katarina feeling crushed and shamed. In this context, Colman argues:

> All sexuality is a form of "enactment" – the issue is the difference between enactments that are concrete and shut down meaning and those that allow for different meanings and have the quality of playfulness that is characteristic of creative, living metaphors.
>
> (Colman, 2009, p. 42)

Colman's perspective is consonant with Winnicott's (1988) description of psychotherapy as being a form of playing – that the initial task of the therapist is to enable the patient to play and become creative. As Phillips (1988) points out, "This means, of course, that the analyst has to be able to play as well" (p. 142). Moreover, in terms of learning from, and being changed by, the patient (Aron, 1996; Casement, 1990), Katarina had chided me in the past on my having made a particularly clumsy transference interpretation, telling me in no uncertain terms: "Paul, not everything's a bloody transference, you know." In doing so, Katarina was reminding me that we have a real relationship, too.

Over and above these considerations, the discerning reader will have noted that my self-disclosure stopped well short of explicitly revealing to Katarina whether or not I was attracted to her sexually. In my view, such self-revelation, regardless of whether it was in the affirmative or non-affirmative, would have been too radical and concrete, characterised by "therapeutic excess" (Mills, 2012) and the mode of psychic equivalence, rather than the pretend mode (I return to this below). Given this, it would have robbed the interaction of its playful "as if" quality.

As I am sure the reader will appreciate, sensitivity to Katarina's feelings, together with the preservation of a playful ambiguity, preclude me from disclosing here whether or not I desired her sexually. Although it may be argued that this was implicit in my "romantic weekend" intervention, I would caution against drawing too literal or concrete a conclusion from this playful comment. That said, and particularly in the light of Gabbard and Hobday's (2012) findings, as discussed above, I think we have to accept that, at times, we are all vulnerable to self-deception and attempts to defeat and triumph over our superego. In recognition of this, I would emphasise the importance of regular, ongoing supervision, as I note in drawing this paper to a conclusion. This notwithstanding, in terms of therapeutic action, I would argue that the salient clinical issue in this instance is that this particular intervention led to an emotionally meaningful "moment of meeting" (Boston Change Process Study Group, 2010) (see discussion below).

More generally, my decision to self-disclose in the way that I did needs to be considered in the context of the unique intersubjective relationship that emerged between Katarina and me. Almost from the start, this was robust, characterised by a feisty struggle about boundaries, but also by emotional honesty, humour, playfulness, and irony. With any other patient, even given similar clinical issues, what emerges, in terms of the "analytic third" (Aron, 2008; Benjamin, 2004; Ogden, 2004) and "reciprocal mutual influence" (Beebe & Lachmann, 2002), would again be unique to that particular relationship, and thus would inevitably be engaged with in a very different way. In other words, from a relational perspective, there is no standard technical way of intervening with a patient's sexuality (Maroda, 2010; Mitchell, 2000).

From the perspective of the Boston Change Process Study Group (2010), much of the interaction between me and Katarina may be said to have taken place in the nonverbal, implicit/enactive domain. As discussed above, intersubjective experience in this domain is changed by the emergence of "now moments" and "moments of meeting" in a context of destabilisation and perturbation. Stern (2004) emphasises that anxiety on the part of the therapist may preclude engagement in "now moments" with the result that the opportunity for change at a key moment is lost. I would suggest that what unfolded between me and Katarina in the session in question resulted in a "now moment", culminating in a "moment of meeting" following my playful boundary setting comment: "It's such a damned shame I'm your therapist, isn't it?"

Thus, while Katarina's initial experience of me in the present was shaped by implicit memories and masochistic expectations of rejection and humiliation, as encoded in an archaic representational model from her silent past, the "moment of meeting" brought our respective implicit relational knowing into a changed state of "intersubjective consciousness". This was facilitated by my use of humour (Lemma, 2000) and by the verbal expression of my thoughts and fantasies, which, in combination with ongoing moment-to-moment mutual regulation in the implicit domain (Beebe et al., 2005), cleared the way for Katarina to use me as her therapist, deepened our therapeutic relationship and, paradoxically, generated a mutual sense of trust and safety for our work together to continue.

From this developmental perspective, it may be argued that Katarina's sexuality was merely the vehicle for the expression of her subjectivity and concomitant affective states, which posed a particular relational challenge, and which required an authentic emotional response. This aspect of the relational process may, again, be seen as a nuanced example of Freud's concept of *Nachträglichkeit*, as previously noted.

In terms of Liotti's (1999) thinking, as discussed above, it may be said that Katarina initially "chose" to activate the sexual motivational system in her interaction with me in this particular encounter. This served to inhibit the attachment system where her real pain lies, in terms of loss, rejection and abandonment. More generally, I think that Katarina's cumulative attachment trauma compromised the interrelated developmental accomplishments of affect regulation and mentalisation. These interlinked capacities provide the developmental basis for emotional connectedness or intersubjective relatedness. To my mind, my playful, improvisatory response to Katarina's plea for us to become intimately, even sexually, involved helped to shift the encounter from a non-reflective, essentially disconnected, style of interacting characterised by the concrete mode of "psychic equivalence", to a reflective, intersubjective form of relating characterised by creative play in the "pretend mode" (Fonagy, 2008b; Fonagy et al., 2002; Fonagy & Target, 1996).

Moreover, although my playful self-disclosure was risky, I think that it was not only what I said but also the way that I said it that proved therapeutic. By this, I mean that my tone of voice, rhythmic cadences, and facial expression in response to my observations of Katarina's expressive display all created a cross-modal match with her psychobiological state (Beebe et al., 2005; Colman, 2009; Stern, 1985). As informed by mother-infant developmental studies and neuroscience findings relating to the mirror neuron system (Gallese, 2009), the implicit aspects of the intervention facilitated the repair to the disruption or perturbation that had occurred in our intersubjective relationship as a result of Katarina wanting something from me (an intimate relationship) that I could not give to her. It may, however, be argued that, on an unconscious level, what Katarina actually wanted from me was what, happily, I provided – emotional honesty and a new relational experience within a boundaried relationship.

Taken together, I would argue that these playful interventions facilitated greater integration and freedom of movement between Katarina's attachment behavioural systems or dissociated self-states. Moreover, I would suggest that this particular encounter consisted of a subtle interaction between the nonverbal, implicit domain and the verbal, explicit domain, reflecting Stern's (2004) contention that "making narratives involves not only words, but also direct experiences that are in the implicit domain" (p. 192).

Supervision

Needless to say, these various clinical and ethical issues were discussed in supervision as they arose in the therapeutic relationship. Again, given Gabbard and Hobday's (2012) findings from their work with professionals who have transgressed an ethical boundary, I would stress the importance both of the supervisory relationship and of not becoming isolated in our clinical work, particularly when engaging in a more direct, relational way with a patient's sexuality. As a supervisor myself, I am only too well aware of how intensely unsettling at times a supervisee can find the relational challenges of sexuality in the consulting room. This is particularly so when the emergent sexual attraction and desire is mutual and it is the first time the supervisee has experienced "lustful love" in their clinical practice. Helping the supervisee to contain their anxiety, retain the analytic role and function, and find the language to talk to the patient about this aspect of the therapeutic relationship not only facilitates the process of change, but also helps to preclude the premature ending of the therapy, on the one hand, and the violation of a sexual boundary, on the other hand.

Conclusion

In the intervening years of therapy, there was a marked lessening in both Katarina's fear that I would die or abandon her in some way and in her bids for an intimate relationship. As noted above, I would see these two clinical issues as inextricably linked. As Katarina became more able to trust in my emotional availability, so her anxious, preoccupied attachment behaviour, characterised by a clinging hyper-vigilance and tendency to sexualise relationships, receded into the background.

While I am not arguing that these changes were the direct result of my self-disclosure in response to Katarina's bids for a sexual relationship, I would suggest they indicated that the emotional quality of our therapeutic relationship, together with the co-construction of a meaningful narrative, helped to facilitate an adaptive organisation of her state of mind in respect of attachment trauma. It also seemed to enhance her sense of self-organisation and self-agency (Knox, 2011), as reflected by the fact that Katarina felt able to embark on a lengthy and arduous professional training in a field of her own choosing. Moreover, I would contend that the evident improvement in her self-coherence and capacities for affect regulation and mentalisation confirms the respective findings of Roth and Fonagy (1996), Schore (1994), Stern et al. (1998), and Shedler (2010), viz., that the interactive emotion-transacting aspect of the therapeutic relationship is the main mechanism of intrapsychic change. Indeed, Gabbard and Hobday (2012) cite findings showing that "a solid therapeutic alliance" has "consistently been found to be the best predictor of outcome in psychotherapy research" (p. 246).

These findings accord with my clinical experience of some 30 years in both a forensic setting and private practice. From a neuroscience perspective, the inherent demands and challenges of the therapeutic relationship create new neural connections which, in attachment terms, are conceptualised as second order self-other representational models and the attainment of "earned security" (Cozolino, 2002, 2006; Diamond & Kernberg, 2008; Fonagy et al., 1995; Fonagy, 1999; Hesse, 1999; Holmes, 2010; Levy et al., 2006; Renn, 2012).

This chapter has argued that working with sexuality in the consulting room demands neither avoidance nor permissiveness, but rather a clinical stance grounded in sustained reflection, relational responsibility, and a commitment to keeping experience thinkable. The challenges posed by sexuality illuminate the broader principles that govern relational work: the necessity of recognition, the risks of mutual influence, the imperative of ethical vigilance, and the transformative potential of moments of meeting when these can be held within a secure and reflective therapeutic frame.

The next chapter turns to the far edge of relational breakdown – psychosis and severe anxiety – showing how even these extreme states can be understood through the same relational-neurodevelopmental lens.

Acknowledgement

This chapter is adapted from "Moments of Meeting: The Relational Challenges of Sexuality in the Consulting Room", *BJP*, 29(2) (May 2013), pp. 135–153.

References

Aron, L. (1996). *A meeting of minds: Mutuality in psychoanalysis*. Hillsdale, NJ: Analytic Press.

Aron, L. (2008). Relational psychoanalysis: Evolution of theory, implications for practice. In S. Akhtar (ed.), *Regarding others: Clinical and theoretical essays on otherness* (pp. 75–100). London: Karnac Books.

Beebe, B. & Lachmann, F. M. (2002). *Infant research and adult treatment: Co-constructing interactions*. Hillsdale, NJ: Analytic Press.

Beebe, B., Knoblauch, S., Rustin, J. & Sorter, D. (2005). *Forms of intersubjectivity in infant research and adult treatment: A systems view*. New York: Other Press.

Benjamin, J. (1992). Recognition and destruction: An outline of intersubjectivity. *Psychoanalytic Psychology*, 9, 33–48.

Benjamin, J. (1995). *Like subjects, love objects: Essays on recognition and sexual difference*. New Haven: Yale University Press.

Benjamin, J. (2004). Beyond doer and done to: An intersubjective view of thirdness. *Psychoanalytic Quarterly*, 73, 5–46.

Boston Change Process Study Group. (2010). *Change in psychotherapy: A unifying paradigm*. New York: Norton.

Britton, R. (1997). Making the private public. In I. Ward (ed.), *The presentation of case material in clinical discourse*, pp. 11–28. London: Karnac Books.

Budd, S. (2001). A defence of drives. *Journal of Analytical Psychology*, 46, 553–560.

Casement, P. (1990). *Further learning from the patient*. London: Routledge.

Celenza, A. (2010). The analyst's need and desire. *Psychoanalytic Dialogues*, 20, 60–69.

Celenza, A. & Gabbard, G. O. (2007). Analysts who commit sexual boundary violations. *Journal of the American Psychoanalytic Association*, 55, 159–185.

Colman, A. D. (2009). The enactment of sexuality in clinical work. *Psychoanalytic Dialogues*, 19, 1–21.

Cozolino, L. J. (2002). *The neuroscience of psychotherapy: Building and rebuilding the human brain*. New York: Norton.

Diamond, D. & Kernberg, O. F. (2008). Attachment-based perspectives on psychotherapy. *Journal of the American Psychoanalytic Association*, 56, 739–775.

Feltham, C. (2007). *What's wrong with counselling and therapy?* London: Sage.

Fonagy, P. (1999). Memory and therapeutic action. *International Journal of Psychoanalysis*, 80, 215–223.

Fonagy, P. (2008a). The mentalisation-focused approach to social development. In F. N. Busch (ed.), *Mentalisation: Theoretical considerations, research findings, and clinical implications* (pp. 3–56). Hove: Analytic Press.

Fonagy, P. (2008b). A genuinely developmental theory of sexual enjoyment and its implications for psychoanalytic technique. *Journal of the American Psychoanalytic Association*, 56, 11–36.

Fonagy, P., Gergely, G., Jurist, E. & Target, M. (2002). *Affect regulation, mentalization, and the development of the self*. New York: Other Press.

Fonagy, P., Steele, M., Steele, H., Leigh, T., Kennedy, R. & Mattoon, G. (1995). Attachment, the reflective self, and borderline states: The predictive specificity of the Adult Attachment Interview and pathological emotional development. In S. Goldberg, R. Muir & J. Kerr (eds), *Attachment theory: Social, developmental and clinical perspectives* (pp. 233–278). Hillsdale, NJ: Analytic Press.

Fonagy, P. & Target, M. (1996). Playing with reality: I. Theory of mind and the normal development of psychic reality. *International Journal of Psychoanalysis, 77* (2), 217–233.

Friedman, R. (2010). The analyst's emotional responses. *Psychoanalytic Quarterly,* 79, 1–29.

Gabbard, G. O. (1996). *Love and hate in the analytic setting*. Northvale, NJ: Jason Aronson.

Gabbard, G. O. & Hobday, G. S. (2012). A psychoanalytic perspective on ethics, self-deception and the corrupt physician. *British Journal of Psychotherapy,* 28(2), 235–248.

Gabbard, G. O. & Lester, E. P. (1995). *Boundaries and boundary violations in psychoanalysis*. New York: Basic Books.

Gallese, V. (2009). The two sides of mimesis: Girard's mimetic theory, embodied simulation, and social identification. *Journal of Consciousness Studies,* 16, 21–44.

Green, A. (1996). Has sexuality anything to do with psychoanalysis? *International Journal of Psychoanalysis, 77,* 871–883.

Harding, C. (2001). Sexuality and the new paradigm. *Journal of Analytical Psychology,* 46, 527–546.

Hesse, E. (1999). The adult attachment interview: Historical and current perspectives. In J. Cassidy & P. R. Shaver (eds), *Handbook of attachment: Theory, research, and clinical applications* (pp. 395–433). New York: Guilford Press.

Holmes, J. (2007). Notes on sexuality and attachment. *Attachment & Human Development,* 9, 1–10.

Holmes, J. (2010). *Exploring in security: Towards an attachment-informed psychoanalytic psychotherapy*. London: Routledge.

Knox, J. (2011). *Self-agency in psychotherapy: Attachment, autonomy and intimacy.* New York: Norton.

Lemma, A. (2000). *Humour on the couch: Exploring humour in psychotherapy and everyday life*. London: Whurr Publishers.

Levy, K. N., Meehan, K. B., Kelly, K. M., Reynoso, J. S., Weber, M., Clarkin, J. F. & Kernberg, O. F. (2006). Change in attachment patterns and reflective function in a randomized controlled trial of transference-focused psychotherapy for borderline personality disorder. *Journal of Consulting and Clinical Psychology,* 74, 1027–1040.

Lichtenberg, J. D. (2007). Sexuality and attachment across the divide of shame. *Psychoanalytic Inquiry,* 27, 434–447.

Lichtenberg, J. D. (2008). Sensuality and sexuality. *Psychoanalytic Inquiry,* 28, 1–15.

Liotti, G. (1999). Disorganized attachment, dissociation and dissociative disorders. *Dissociation,* 12, 171–183.

Litowitz, B. (2002). Sexuality and textuality. *Journal of the American Psychoanalytic Association,* 50, 171–198.

Mann, D. (1997). *Psychotherapy: An erotic relationship*. London: Routledge.

Maroda, K. J. (2010). *Psychodynamic techniques: Working with emotion in the therapeutic relationship*. New York: Guilford Press.

Martin, P., Godfrey, E. & Meekums, B. (2011). Sexuality in the therapeutic relationship. *Counselling and Psychotherapy Research,* 11, 1–10.

Mills, J. (2012). The ethics of disclosure in psychoanalysis. *American Journal of Psychotherapy,* 66, 311–337.

Mitchell, S. A. (1988). *Relational concepts in psychoanalysis.* Cambridge, MA: Harvard University Press.

Mitchell, S. A. (1997). *Influence and autonomy in psychoanalysis*. Hillsdale, NJ: Analytic Press.

Mitchell, S. A. (2000). *Relationality: From attachment to intersubjectivity*. Hillsdale, NJ: Analytic Press.

Ogden, T. H. (2004). The analytic third: Implications for psychoanalytic theory and technique. *Psychoanalytic Quarterly*, 73(1), 167–195.

Phillips, A. (1988). *Winnicott*. London: Fontana Press.

Renn, P. (2012). *The silent past and the invisible present: Memory, trauma, and representation in psychotherapy*. New York: Routledge.

Renn, P. (2013). Moments of meeting: The relational challenges of sexuality in the consulting room. *British Journal of Psychotherapy*, 29(2), 135–153.

Ringstrom, P. (2008). Improvisation and the therapeutic relationship. *Psychoanalytic Inquiry*, 28, 1–21.

Rodgers, B. (2011). Sexual attraction in therapy. *Psychotherapy*, 48, 265–275.

Roth, A. & Fonagy, P. (1996). *What works for whom? A critical review of psychotherapy research*. New York: Guilford Press.

Schore, A. N. (1994). *Affect regulation and the origin of the self*. Hillsdale, NJ: Lawrence Erlbaum Associates.

Shedler, J. (2010). The efficacy of psychodynamic psychotherapy. *American Psychologist*, 65, 98–109.

Stein, R. (1998). The poignant, the excessive and the enigmatic in sexuality. *International Journal of Psychoanalysis*, 79, 253–268.

Stern, D. N. (1985). *The interpersonal world of the infant*. New York: Basic Books.

Stern, D. N. (2004). *The present moment in psychotherapy and everyday life*. New York: Norton.

Stern, D. N., Sander, L. W., Nahum, J. P., Harrison, A. M., Lyons-Ruth, K., Morgan, A. C., Bruschweiler-Stern, N. & Tronick, E. Z. (1998). The process of therapeutic change involving implicit knowledge: Some implications of developmental observations for adult psychotherapy. *Infant Mental Health Journal*, 19(3), 300–308.

Target, M. (2007). Sexuality and attachment. *Psychoanalytic Inquiry*, 27, 448–464.

Tyson, P. (2002). The challenges of psychoanalytic developmental theory. *Journal of the American Psychoanalytic Association*, 50(1), 19–52.

Winnicott, D. W. (1965). Communicating and not communicating leading to a study of certain opposites. In *The Maturational Processes and the Facilitating Environment* (pp. 179–192). London: Hogarth Press.

Winnicott, D. W. (1988). *Human nature*. London: Free Association Books.

12 Relational Perspectives on Psychosis and Anxiety

Retrospective Reflection

This chapter originated as a teaching programme developed for fourth-year psychotherapy trainees at a time when psychosis occupied a marginal position within much psychoanalytic training and was frequently regarded as either diagnostically fixed or analytically inaccessible. My intention at that time was to provide a relationally grounded framework through which trainees might begin to engage with psychosis and severe anxiety without resorting to premature categorisation or defensive theoretical retreat. The emphasis was therefore on exposing students to a range of relational, developmental, and socio-political perspectives capable of restoring meaning to states of mind often experienced as terrifying, opaque, or beyond understanding.

In the years since this material was first taught, my thinking has increasingly coalesced around the concept of cumulative relational trauma as a central organising principle in psychological development and breakdown. Re-reading this chapter in that light, it is striking how much it already anticipates a developmental and neurobiological understanding of psychosis as an extreme outcome of repeated failures of affect regulation, attachment-mediated containment, and intersubjective recognition. What was once presented primarily as a pluralistic map can now be understood as pointing towards a more integrated relational-neurodevelopmental account.

In revising the chapter for this volume, I have therefore sought not to replace its original teaching purpose, but to bring its underlying coherence more clearly into view. Psychosis and severe anxiety are approached here not as exceptional pathologies but as extreme states within a continuum of human response to overwhelming relational threat. In this sense, the chapter occupies a pivotal position in the book: it tests the reach of the model at its most extreme clinical edge and prepares the ground for the more explicit theoretical synthesis that follows.

DOI: 10.4324/9781003789727-16

Psychosis, Anxiety, and Cumulative Relational Trauma

This chapter approaches psychosis and severe anxiety not as discrete diagnostic entities but as extreme developmental outcomes of cumulative relational trauma. From a relational-neurodevelopmental perspective, psychotic states are understood as organised responses to overwhelming danger, arising when early affect regulation, attachment-mediated containment, and the capacity to differentiate inner from outer reality have been repeatedly compromised. Psychosis, in this sense, does not sit outside ordinary human development but represents a limit condition of processes continuous with those shaping less extreme forms of psychological suffering.

Object relations theorists have long described psychotic states in terms of catastrophic experiences of futility, terror, and powerlessness. The accompanying disintegration of subjectivity or sense of an embodied self is lived as pervasive external threat, internal persecution, and intense oscillations between isolation and engulfment. Such states are often marked by a collapse in the capacity to discriminate between "me" and "not-me", self and other. Winnicott described this as the perpetual human task of keeping inner and outer realities separate yet interrelated (Winnicott, 1974). From a cumulative trauma perspective, the breakdown of this task reflects not sudden collapse but the end point of repeated failures in relational holding and recognition.

Psychosis confronts clinicians with the problem of consensual meaning. Delusion has traditionally been taken as the hallmark of madness, raising the question of how one is to understand experience in the absence of a shared reality. Yet while overt psychosis affects a minority of individuals, madness remains an implicit thread in social and political discourse, often invoked to symbolise destructiveness, violence, or evil. As Eigen (1986) observed, psychosis takes us to the edge of what is possible to experience, and yet it has remained something of a "Cinderella" within psychoanalysis.

Anxiety as Signal Affect and Developmental Bridge

A central contention of this chapter is that anxiety provides the developmental bridge between cumulative relational trauma and psychotic breakdown. Anxiety may be understood as the primary emotional signal of perceived danger within attachment relationships. Under conditions of sufficient attuned caregiving, anxiety mobilises attachment, draws the caregiver closer, and is metabolised through interactive regulation. In such contexts, anxiety remains representable and thinkable.

Where caregiving is misattuned, frightening, intrusive, or withdrawn, anxiety ceases to function as a signal and instead becomes a disorganising force. Repeated failures of containment leave anxiety unregulated, shorn of shared experience, and increasingly intolerable. From this point, defensive operations such as dissociation, hypervigilance, and perceptual distortion emerge as adaptive responses. Psychosis may often reflect what occurs when these defences are no longer sufficient to contain terror and when anxiety overwhelms the psyche's capacity for integration.

Seen in this light, psychosis is not the absence of anxiety but its transformation. Panic becomes persecution; hypervigilance becomes paranoia; unmentalised affect crystallises into delusional meaning. This formulation allows psychosis and severe anxiety to be located along a single developmental continuum rather than as qualitatively distinct conditions (Schore, 2003; Fonagy et al., 2002).

Delusion as Meaning Under Siege

From a relational perspective, delusions may be understood not as meaningless products of disordered thought but as attempts to preserve coherence under conditions of overwhelming relational threat. Stolorow, Brandchaft, and Atwood described delusions as communications that the self is crumbling and struggling to hold together – a last stop before the abyss (Stolorow et al., 1987). Such phenomena cannot be understood apart from the intersubjective contexts in which they arise and recede.

Laing's concept of ontological insecurity similarly emphasised the terror of annihilation that arises when the self cannot rely on others as sources of safety. For Laing, what is called psychosis may sometimes represent the sudden collapse of a "false self" organisation behind which the individual has been "playing at being sane" (Laing, 1990 [1959]). Delusional accounts, far from being absurd, often acquire intelligibility when situated within familial and social contexts characterised by contradictory demands and power asymmetries (Laing & Esterson, 1964).

From a narrative standpoint, delusions may be understood as creative attributions of meaning to experiences of disintegration. Roberts argued that delusional narratives arise from the healthy part of the person attempting to organise anomalous experience and compensate for losses and traumas that are too painful to acknowledge directly (Roberts, 1999). Taken together, these perspectives suggest that delusion is not the opposite of meaning but meaning under siege – an effort to impose coherence where relational containment has failed.

Searles's work offers a further deepening of this view by highlighting how psychotic experience emerges within a field of unbearable interpersonal pressure. In his account of "the effort to drive the other person crazy", Searles (1993) described how psychotic communication often reflects an attempt to manage relational environments that are so incoherent or traumatising they threaten the very continuity of the self. His clinical observations underscore the extent to which delusional meaning-making arises not in isolation but in response to overwhelming relational contradictions – an effort to preserve psychic organisation when the boundaries between self and other have been repeatedly destabilised. In a similar way to Stolorow et al. (1987), Searles's perspective emphasises that delusions need to be understood in the intersubjective contexts in which they develop. It also reinforces the view of psychosis as an organised response to cumulative relational trauma rather than a departure from human intelligibility.

Developmental and Neurobiological Organisation

Developmental research lends strong support to the view that psychosis has its origins in early relational failure. Mahler and Furer (1967) described childhood psychosis in terms of a failure of individuation, often associated with caregiving relationships that were excessively intrusive or parasitic. Daniel Stern (1985) later conceptualised such failures as disturbances in affect attunement, resulting in deficits in the capacity to share emotional and intentional states within intersubjective space.

Contemporary attachment research and developmental neuroscience have further elucidated how cumulative relational trauma becomes organised in mind and brain. Disorganised attachment, unresolved caregiver trauma, and chronic misattunement compromise the development of affect regulation and the monitoring of internal states of consciousness (Main & Hesse, 1990; Schore, 2003). Fonagy and colleagues have shown how failures of reflective functioning leave inner experience barren, terrifying, and unrepresentable, laying the groundwork for later fragmentation under stress (Fonagy et al., 2002).

Neurobiological findings indicating that early stress alters neural development parallel those observed in individuals diagnosed with schizophrenia, post-traumatic stress disorder, and dissociative disorders. These findings do not replace psychoanalytic understanding but provide a relational-neurodevelopmental account of how trauma becomes biologically embedded.

Trauma, Dissociation, and Diagnostic Collapse

Research on trauma and dissociation increasingly challenges rigid diagnostic boundaries between psychosis, post-traumatic stress disorder, dissociative disorders, and severe personality disturbance. Studies of combat veterans, survivors of abuse, and individuals exposed to chronic relational trauma reveal substantial overlap in symptomatology, including hypervigilance, intrusive imagery, dissociation, and paranoid ideation (Read et al., 2004).

From this perspective, dissociation and psychosis may be understood as adaptive responses to overwhelming threat rather than as indicators of discrete disease entities. Diagnostic distinctions often obscure the developmental continuity linking early relational trauma to later breakdown. It may therefore be more productive to conceptualise these conditions as variations within a long-term process initiated by adaptive responses to aversive environments rather than as categorically distinct disorders.

Power, Racism, and Institutional Trauma

Cumulative relational trauma is not confined to early caregiving environments but may be enacted and sustained at institutional and societal levels. The disproportionate diagnosis of psychosis among Black and minority ethnic communities has been linked to experiences of racism, social exclusion, and coercive psychiatric practices (Fernando, 1999). Fanon (1967) understood racism as psychic trauma, while subsequent writers have emphasised the intergenerational impact of historical oppression and slavery on mental health.

Labelling theory further illuminates how social power shapes psychiatric diagnosis and response. Once labelled, individuals may become trapped within deviant identities that reinforce alienation and despair. From a relational perspective, institutional racism and coercive care constitute chronic relational trauma, eliciting states of fear, mistrust, and fragmentation that may themselves precipitate psychotic experience.

Clinical and Ethical Implications

Relational perspectives have contributed to a re-evaluation of the traditional exclusion of psychotic individuals from psychoanalytic treatment. Work at this clinical edge confronts the analyst with terror, dread, and the limits of their own capacity for containment. As noted in Chapter 8, Mitchell (1993) observed that pseudo-normality may be the central clinical problem of our time. This echoes Winnicott's suggestion that a life confined solely to sanity is itself an impoverished one.

Engaging psychosis relationally requires the therapist to tolerate proximity to madness without retreating into defensive objectification or premature normalisation. It demands a willingness to remain in contact with unmentalised affect and to recognise the mutual vulnerability of the analytic encounter. In this sense, work with psychosis returns psychoanalysis to its ethical foundations: the commitment to meaning, relationship, and hope in the face of terror.

From the perspective developed across this volume, psychosis and severe anxiety are best understood as extreme expressions of cumulative relational trauma, organised developmentally and transmitted intergenerationally. Relational psychoanalysis remains uniquely placed to work at this limit precisely because it refuses to abandon relationship where relationship has most profoundly failed. These clinical extremes highlight the need for an integrative model capable of holding relational, developmental, and neurobiological processes together. Chapter 14 outlines such a model.

References

Eigen, M. (1986). *The psychotic core*. Northvale, NJ: Jason Aronson.
Fanon, F. (1967). *Black skin, white masks*. New York: Grove Press.

Fernando, S. (1999). Race in the construction of dangerousness. Paper presented at the Bowlby Memorial Lecture, London.

Fonagy, P., Gergely, G., Jurist, E. & Target, M. (2002). *Affect regulation, mentalization, and the development of the self*. New York: Other Press.

Laing, R. D. (1990 [1959]). *The divided self*. Harmondsworth: Penguin.

Laing, R. D. & Esterson, A. (1964). *Sanity, madness and the family*. London: Penguin.

Mahler, M. S. & Furer, M. (1967). On human symbiosis and the vicissitudes of individuation: Infantile psychosis. *Journal of the American Psychoanalytic Association*, 15, 740–753.

Main, M. & Hesse, E. (1990). Parents' unresolved traumatic experiences are related to infant disorganized attachment status. In M. Greenberg, D. Cicchetti & E. Cummings (eds), *Attachment in the preschool years* (pp. 161–182). Chicago: University of Chicago Press.

Mitchell, S. A. (1993). *Hope and dread in psychoanalysis*. New York: Basic Books.

Read, J., Goodman, L., Morrison, A. P., Ross, C. A. & Aderhold, V. (2004). Childhood trauma, loss and stress. In J. Read, L. R. Mosher & R. P. Bentall (eds), *Models of madness* (pp. 223–252). London: Routledge.

Roberts, G. (1999). The rehabilitation of rehabilitation: A narrative approach to psychosis. In G. Roberts & J. Holmes (eds), *Healing stories* (pp. 152–180). Oxford: Oxford University Press.

Schore, A. N. (2003). *Affect dysregulation and disorders of the self*. New York: Norton.

Searles, H. (1993). The effort to drive the other person crazy: An element in the aetiology and psychotherapy of schizophrenia. In H. Searles, *Collected papers on schizophrenia and related subjects* (pp. 284–303). Madison, CT: International Universities Press.

Stern, D. N. (1985). *The interpersonal world of the infant*. New York: Basic Books.

Stolorow, R. D., Brandchaft, B. & Atwood, G. E. (1987). *Psychoanalytic treatment: An intersubjective approach*. Hillsdale, NJ: Analytic Press.

Winnicott, D. W. (1974). Fear of breakdown. *International Review of Psychoanalysis*, 1, 103–107.

13 Working with the Patient's Everyday Relational World

Procedural Templates, Enactment, and the Site of Change

Retrospective Reflection

Looking back on the evolution of this chapter, I am struck by how long it took me to articulate explicitly something that has been quietly shaping my clinical work for many years. The consulting room remains a vital space, but it is not the only one. The patient's everyday relational world is where the past becomes present, where procedural templates are enacted, and where new possibilities can take root.

In revisiting Mitchell's work with Connie, I found myself reflecting not only on his clinical courage but also on my own hesitations. There has long been a sense, sometimes subtle, sometimes more insistent, that focusing on everyday relationships risks straying from the sanctified terrain of transference, or that it might be judged as insufficiently analytic. Britton's notion of "publication anxiety" (Britton, 1997 *, p. 14) resonates here: the fear of stepping outside established boundaries and being quietly, or not so quietly, sanctioned for it.*

Yet the more I wrote, the clearer it became that this dimension is not peripheral but central. It is the bridge between the silent past and the invisible present. It is where trauma is repeated and where healing is consolidated. And it is where the analytic project, at its best, becomes woven into the fabric of a patient's lived life. What shifted for me was the recognition that the most meaningful changes my patients described were occurring not in the consulting room but in their everyday intimate relationships.

If this chapter helps legitimise that work, or gives clinicians permission to follow their patients into the relational spaces that matter most, then it has earned its place in the volume.

Introduction

Across this volume, I have explored how trauma, attachment, implicit memory, and relational configurations shape the inner world and its enactments. One theme, however, has remained somewhat implicit: that the consulting room, while central, is not the only arena in which therapeutic

DOI: 10.4324/9781003789727-17

change takes place. This perspective is not without precedent. Freud (1912) stressed that transference is not confined to the consulting room but is a ubiquitous feature of mental life, continuously shaping the patient's everyday relationships. He elaborated this view more explicitly in later works such as the *Introductory Lectures* (Freud, 1916–1917). This early recognition of transference as a pervasive phenomenon anticipates later relational perspectives that view everyday interactions as continuous with analytic process. Freud's observation, then, underscores that the patient's everyday relationships are not external to analytic work but continuous with the analytic field itself.

It follows that a significant proportion of the work of transformation occurs in the patient's everyday relational life – the site where procedural templates are most vividly enacted in small but telling moments – a partner's sigh, a colleague's silence, a child's withdrawal. Such moments often indicate the sudden activation of an archaic template. Engagement with such moments provides powerful opportunities for the modification of maladaptive procedural ways of relating.

This chapter brings that dimension into clearer focus. It grows out of a commentary I wrote on Paul Wachtel's (2017) paper on relationality in everyday life, and it uses that discussion as a springboard to articulate more explicitly how everyday relationships function as the crucible in which the inner world is continually recreated.

Theoretical Background: Relational Multiplicity and Everyday Life

Wachtel (2017) argues that relational psychoanalysis has tended to underplay the patient's wider relational system. As I wrote in my commentary, "I wholeheartedly agree with and endorse Wachtel's emphasis on the therapeutic benefit of working with the patient's wider relational system, as experienced in his or her everyday life" (Renn, 2017, p. 522). This emphasis aligns with the relational tradition's longstanding interest in mutual influence, enactment, and co-constructed meaning. Just as the analytic field is co-constructed, so too is the patient's everyday world a shifting matrix of meanings, expectations, and enactments.

Yet I also noted a tension. Wachtel's passionate tone risked sounding prescriptive in a field that values pluralism and tentativeness. Mitchell (1993) captured this ethos when he wrote that "meaning lends itself to multiple understandings ... human experience is fundamentally ambiguous" (p. 58). The relational tradition is not a school with fixed doctrines but a multiplicity of perspectives, each shaped by the analyst's own sensibility.

Still, the core of Wachtel's argument is difficult to ignore. The inner world is not a sealed chamber but a dynamic system continually shaped by daily relational transactions. These transactions are not peripheral to analytic work; they are central to it.

Mitchell's Evolving Thinking: From Developmental Tilt to Implicit Knowing

Mitchell's early critique of the "developmental tilt" (Mitchell, 1988) already contained the seeds of a more complex understanding of repetition. Even then, he acknowledged the significance of early experience but insisted that repetition should be understood as "a vehicle for comprehending the meaning of current relationships" (p. 151).

By the late 1990s, influenced by Beatrice Beebe, Daniel Stern, and the Boston Change Process Study Group, Mitchell increasingly emphasised implicit relational knowing – "procedural knowledge" that illuminates "what is actually going on in the patient's life" (Mitchell, 2000, p. 61). This shift had profound clinical implications. Mitchell began to view the caregiver-infant relationship as a prototype for adult therapeutic work, not in a regressive sense, but as a model of reciprocal influence, mutual regulation, and co-constructed meaning (Mitchell, 2002). His case study of Connie (Mitchell, 2000) is a vivid illustration of this evolution.

Repetition and Transformation in Connie's Relationship with Her Husband

Connie's mother was killed in a car accident when Connie was five years old. Her father was unable to help her and her older brother mourn the loss, which was never spoken about. Instead, he sent both of them away to separate boarding schools. Connie would see her father at weekends, but seven years were to elapse before she was allowed to live at home again on a regular basis. Connie experienced her father as extremely brittle throughout her childhood and was careful not to burden him with her own needs.

Connie commenced a psychotherapy in her mid-30s, during which she worked on the consequences of her early loss. Although the therapy was quite successful, the sadness that had blighted her whole life remained, becoming more severe when she married in her late 30s and had a son. She entered analysis with Mitchell in her mid-40s, by which time the boy was five years old. He had intense separation anxiety and Connie feared that her tragic early life was negatively impacting him. She had a distinct sense of being merged with both him and her mother in some way: That she was part of them and they were part of her. Her work with Mitchell at this stage focused on helping her to contain experiences of both union and separation from her son, and to loosen the unconscious tie to her dead mother.

Despite this progress, Connie was almost paralysed by painful feelings. She experienced her sadness as a "bottomless pit" and feared that the analysis would stir up even more distressing losses. Mitchell (2000) began to suspect that "there was something in the way Connie organized her current experiences that contributed to regenerating her sadness; that her feelings reflected something she was giving up in the present as much as something she had lost in the past" (p. 93). This seemed to be founded "on a chronic sense of sadness and of something missing" (p. 93).

This "prototypical" way of organising her experience in general, and sadness in particular, was most apparent in her relationship with her husband. He was a rather self-absorbed man and not readily emotionally available to Connie. As with her father, and redolent of Winnicott's (1987) "false self", Connie had seamlessly adapted to what was intimately available from her husband. Indeed, she had decided long ago that he was "simply unavailable to meet her emotional needs, and so had stopped even being aware of having any such needs vis-à-vis him" (p. 98).

As the analysis continued, Connie reported becoming increasingly aware of a chronic sense of grievance against her husband because he continually took her for granted. Her resentment would mount up and she would then angrily express her feelings to him, leaving him feeling attacked in an inappropriately intense way. Typically, Connie would end up apologising to him for her behaviour. Mitchell (2000) "got interested in the way Connie presented her concerns to her husband" (p. 99), and the sessions "primarily explored various facets of her relationship with her husband" (p. 100). Connie's distress centred on her sense that "she did not exist for him, as if she had no presence in his mind … and it was her chronic, pervasive sense of isolation that contributed to her perpetual sadness" (p. 99). Thus, she ended up "trapped in her familiar but sad solitude" (p. 99).

Mitchell (2000) suggested to Connie alternative ways of discussing her feelings with her husband – that she express how much "she valued a feeling of connection with him, that his acting as if he was unaware of the impact of his behavior on her made her feel as if she had no place in his mind" (p. 99). In doing so, Mitchell acknowledged that such a way of intervening "is not generally considered within the bounds of traditional analytic technique" (p. 100). For Connie, however, the thought of actively expressing her needs in this way both exhilarated and frightened her. "She feared that anyone becoming aware of her need for them would likely feel burdened and abandon her" (p. 100). This notwithstanding, as time went on she became more adept at expressing her own needs to her husband, as well as feeling a certain freedom from his need of her. In turn, he came out of his self-absorption with work and made himself more intimately available to her.

Discussion: Relational Cycles and the Plasticity of Change

Connie's case illustrates that trauma and attachment patterns are not merely static internal structures but dynamic relational processes enacted within ongoing interpersonal exchanges (Tolmacz, 2009). As Wachtel (2017) emphasises in his cyclical psychodynamic model, everyday intimate transactions play a critical role in both maintaining and modifying the inner world. These patterns often take the form of self-perpetuating "vicious circles", in which partners inadvertently "recruit accomplices" to sustain familiar, though painful, relational configurations.

One clinically common configuration, consistent with attachment research, involves a partner organised around fears of abandonment paired with a partner who is comparatively uncomfortable with intimacy and inclined towards emotional distance. Such pairings are not incidental but reflect the mutual activation of complementary procedural templates, each reinforcing the other's expectations and defensive strategies (Bowlby, 1979; Dinero et al., 2008; Mikulincer & Shaver, 2007; Simpson, 1990). This pertains in both same-sex and opposite-sex relationships (Mohr, 2008). In Connie's case, her dread of losing her husband contributed to a constricted pattern of self-imposed silence and delayed expression, which in turn elicited his withdrawal and self-absorption. This recursive dynamic not only sustained her own suffering but likely contributed to her son's separation anxiety, illustrating the non-linear, intergenerational transmission of attachment patterns discussed in Chapter 5.

Understanding these dynamics in cyclical terms also clarifies the mechanism of therapeutic change. If maladaptive patterns are maintained through repetition in everyday interactions, then change must involve the introduction of new relational experiences within those same contexts. This is what Wachtel (2017) describes as the transformation of "vicious circles" into "virtuous circles", in which altered responses begin to shift the expectations and behaviours of both partners.

Contemporary neuroscience provides a complementary account of this process, offering a biological perspective on the same relational plasticity. The brain's ongoing plasticity across the lifespan allows for the modification of established patterns of relating through new interpersonal experiences (Cozolino, 2002, 2006). From this perspective, procedural templates and implicit relational knowing are not fixed structures but evolving organisations of experience that can be reshaped through repeated exposure to novel relational contingencies, as explored in Chapter 6. Deliberate experimentation with new ways of expressing needs or responding to others constitutes not merely behavioural change, but the gradual reorganisation of underlying neural and relational patterns.

Mitchell's work with Connie can be understood in precisely these terms. By helping her bring implicit relational knowing into reflective awareness, he enabled her to experiment with new forms of engagement in her marriage. As Connie became more able to articulate her needs directly and without apology, she introduced a new relational demand into the system. Her husband, in turn, was drawn out of his habitual self-absorption and became more emotionally available. Change, therefore, did not occur solely within the consulting room but was realised in the ongoing fabric of Connie's everyday life, where new patterns could be repeatedly enacted, tested, and consolidated.

This perspective has important implications for analytic technique. It suggests that the analyst's task is not only to interpret the patient's experience of relationships, but also to attend closely to how those relationships are actually conducted in everyday life. Moments of misattunement, withdrawal, escalation, and repair become crucial sites of inquiry. At times, this may involve supporting the patient in experimenting with alternative ways of relating, offered not as prescriptive advice, but as opportunities to bring implicit relational knowing into reflective awareness and lived experience.

From an attachment perspective, this approach is consistent with the understanding that internal working models are transmitted and transformed across generations in complex and non-linear ways (Fonagy et al., 2002; Bowlby, 1979, 1988, 1998; Lyons-Ruth & Jacobvitz, 2008). Connie's fear of abandonment, her husband's discomfort with intimacy, and their son's separation anxiety can all be understood as expressions of interlocking relational patterns unfolding across time and context.

Working in this way can evoke the concern that one is departing from "real" analysis (Renn, 2017, p. 528). Mitchell himself acknowledged this tension in his work with Connie. However, such concerns may reflect residual adherence to earlier technical orthodoxies rather than contemporary clinical realities. If procedural templates are most vividly enacted in the patient's everyday relational world, then it follows that this is also where they are most available for transformation (Renn, 2012, 2017; Wachtel, 2008, 2017). Attending to these processes is therefore not a dilution of analytic work, but an extension of it into the domain where change is ultimately lived and sustained.

Conclusion

As Freud (1912, 1916–1917) already noted, transference is lived as much in everyday relationships as within the analytic setting, even if he located its most decisive exploration within the analytic situation. This notwithstanding, his observation of the ubiquitous nature of transference resonates strongly with the clinical material explored here. Indeed, Mitchell's work with Connie offers a compelling framework for attending to the patient's everyday relational world. While the consulting room is the space in which relational patterns are recognised, articulated, and emotionally experienced; everyday relationships are the arena in which those patterns are enacted, tested, and transformed.

From this perspective, therapeutic change depends not only on what is understood within the analytic setting, but also on what can be lived differently beyond it. As patients begin to carry new ways of relating into their daily interactions, implicit relational patterns become available for revision through experience rather than insight alone.

The patient's everyday relational world is therefore not peripheral to analytic work, but central to it. It is here, in the lived fabric of intimate relationships, that the silent past encounters the possibilities of the present – and where new relational futures can begin (Renn, 2012). As I suggested in the retrospective reflection, this dimension of analytic work has long been present, even if unnamed.

Acknowledgement

This chapter is derived, in part, from "Relational Lacunae: Gaps in the Relational Literature and Clinical Practice? Commentary on Paper by Paul Wachtel", *Psychoanalytic Dialogues*, 27(5) (2017), 522–529, doi:10.1080/10481885.2017.1355674.

References

Bowlby, J. (1979). *The making and breaking of affectional bonds*. London: Routledge.

Bowlby, J. (1988). *A secure base: Clinical applications of attachment theory*. London: Routledge.

Bowlby, J. (1998). *Attachment and loss, vol. 3. Loss, sadness and depression*. London: Pimlico.

Britton, R. (1997). Making the private public. In I. Ward (ed.), *The presentation of case material in clinical discourse* (pp. 11–28). London: Karnac.

Cozolino, L. J. (2002). *The neuroscience of psychotherapy: Building and rebuilding the human brain*. New York: Norton.

Cozolino, L. J. (2006). *The neuroscience of human relationships: Attachment and the developing social brain*. New York: Norton.

Dinero, R. E., Conger, R. D., Shaver, P. R., Widaman, K. F. & Larsen-Rife, D. (2008). Influence of family of origin and adult romantic partners on romantic attachment security. *Journal of Family Psychology*, 22(4), 622–632.

Fonagy, P., Gergely, G., Jurist, E. L. & Target, M. (2002). *Affect regulation, mentalization, and the development of the self*. New York: Other Press.

Freud, S. (1912). The dynamics of transference. In J. Strachey (ed.), *The standard edition of the complete psychological works of Sigmund Freud*, vol. 12 (pp. 97–108). London: Hogarth Press.

Freud, S. (1916–1917). Introductory lectures on psycho-analysis. In J. Strachey (ed.), *The standard edition of the complete psychological works of Sigmund Freud*, vol. 15–16. London: Hogarth Press.

Lyons-Ruth, K. & Jacobvitz, D. (2008). Genetic factors, parenting contexts, and developmental transformation. In J. Cassidy & P. R. Shaver (eds), *Handbook of attachment* (2nd ed., pp. 666–697). New York: Guilford Press.

Mikulincer, M. & Shaver, P. R. (2007). *Attachment in adulthood: Structure, dynamics, and change*. New York: Guilford Press.

Mitchell, S. A. (1988). *Relational concepts in psycho-analysis*. Cambridge, MA: Harvard University Press.

Mitchell, S. A. (1993). *Hope and dread in psycho-analysis*. New York: Basic Books.

Mitchell, S. A. (2000). *Relationality: From attachment to intersubjectivity*. Hillsdale, NJ: Analytic Press.

Mitchell, S. A. (2002). *Can love last?*New York: Norton.

Mohr, J. J. (2008). Same-sex romantic attachment. In J. Cassidy & P. R. Shaver (eds), *Handbook of attachment* (2nd ed., pp. 482–502). New York: Guilford Press.

Renn, P. (2012). *The silent past and the invisible present*. New York: Routledge.
Renn, P. (2017). Relational lacunae: Gaps in the relational literature and clinical practice? Commentary on Paper by Paul Wachtel. *Psychoanalytic Dialogues*, 27, 522–529.
Simpson, J. (1990). Influence of attachment styles on romantic relationships. *Journal of Personality and Social Psychology*, 59, 971–980.
Tolmacz, R. (2009). Transference and attachment. In J. H. Obegi & E. Berant (eds), *Attachment theory and research in clinical work with adults* (pp. 269–292). New York: Guilford Press.
Wachtel, P. L. (2008). *Relational theory and the practice of psychotherapy*. New York: Guilford Press.
Wachtel, P. L. (2017). The relationality of everyday life. *Psychoanalytic Dialogues*, 27, 503–521.
Winnicott, D. W. (1987). *The spontaneous gesture*. Cambridge, MA: Harvard University Press.

Part IV

Integration and Future Directions

Introduction to Part IV

Part IV brings the volume full circle. Having traced the developmental foundations of relational life in Part I, examined the dynamics and consequences of cumulative trauma in Part II, and explored clinical process in Part III, this final section gathers these strands into a coherent relational–neurodevelopmental framework. Integration has been both method and aim throughout the book. Rather than reducing one perspective to another, the chapters in this section hold multiple frameworks – psychoanalytic, attachment-informed, developmental, neurobiological, cultural – in productive tension. Part IV makes this integrative stance explicit, showing how these domains illuminate one another without collapsing into eclecticism or theoretical purity.

The four chapters that follow form an integrative meditation, moving from synthesis, to deepening, to critical reflection, and finally to future orientation. Chapter 14 presents a contemporary relational model that brings attachment theory, trauma studies, and neuroscience into dialogue. It illustrates how these perspectives converge around processes of regulation, implicit memory, and relational influence, offering a framework that supports integration without reduction.

Chapter 15 revisits cumulative trauma from the vantage point of the entire volume. No longer simply a concept, cumulative trauma emerges as an organising orientation – one that clarifies how repeated relational disruptions shape expectations, agency, and regulation across development and generations. This chapter also expands the frame to include cultural, systemic, and intergenerational contexts, situating cumulative trauma within broader social structures without resorting to blame or determinism.

Chapter 16 turns to neuroscience, not to extend its findings, but to reflect on its place within relational clinical practice. It affirms the value of neurobiological research in illuminating affect regulation and procedural change, while cautioning against biologisation – the reduction of relational complexity to neural mechanisms. A relational-developmental stance holds

DOI: 10.4324/9781003789727-18

neuroscience as one level of description among many, useful when it deepens clinical understanding but insufficient as an explanatory system.

Chapter 17 (Conclusion) draws these threads together, articulating the stance required for a relational-neurodevelopmental practice grounded in informed uncertainty, relational presence, and developmental understanding. It emphasises that therapeutic change occurs through new relational experience, that cumulative trauma remains the unifying thread of the volume, and that integration requires humility, patience, and sustained engagement. The chapter also considers implications for training, supervision, and the ongoing evolution of clinical theory.

Taken together, these chapters demonstrate that integration is possible without reduction; that cumulative relational trauma provides a coherent organising framework even as its implications deepen; that neuroscience requires thoughtful, critical engagement; and that clinical practice must continue to evolve in dialogue with emerging knowledge. Part IV therefore offers both synthesis and opening. It gathers the conceptual and clinical threads developed across the book while acknowledging that the work remains unfinished. Questions persist, new challenges emerge, and understanding continues to develop.

The animating question of this final section is: where do we go from here? Having traced developmental origins, examined cumulative trauma, and explored clinical process, what stance and vision of practice follow from this integrative journey? The answer offered here is not prescriptive. Instead, it proposes a way of thinking – one that centres the therapeutic relationship as the site of procedural transformation, understands difficulty through the lens of cumulative trauma and adaptation, and holds multiple perspectives in ongoing dialogue. This framework invites clinicians into a continuing conversation about development, trauma, relationship, and change – one that remains open, reflective, and grounded in the lived realities of clinical work.

14 A Contemporary Relational Model

Integrating Attachment, Trauma, and Neuroscience Research

Retrospective Reflection

This chapter represents an early but foundational effort to reconcile the historical tensions between classical psychoanalytic thought and the empirical rigor of attachment theory. At the time of its writing, these two traditions often existed in silos – one focused on the internal world of phantasy, the other on observable proximity-seeking behaviour.

Re-visiting this work today, I see it as the starting point for the volume's broader trajectory towards an integrated relational-neurodevelopmental framework. It establishes how internal working models and representational systems are not just cognitive maps, but encapsulate deeply affective and somatic experience. I have retained the core of the original argument as it illustrates the way in which research in mentalisation and neurobiology began to construct early theoretical bridges, presaging a convergence between these two traditions.

Introduction

Clinical work today unfolds in a landscape shaped by complexity: multilayered histories, intergenerational transmissions, neurobiological sensitivities, and the subtle choreography of two minds meeting in real time. The traditional binaries that once organised our field – mind versus body, intrapsychic versus interpersonal, biology versus relationship – no longer hold. What clinicians need now is a model that reflects how people actually develop, adapt, and heal within living relational systems.

A contemporary relational model begins with a simple but radical premise: the mind is formed, transformed, and continually reorganised in relationship. This is not metaphor but biology, psychology, and lived experience converging. Attachment patterns, stress-response systems, epigenetic markers, and the therapist's own subjectivity all participate in shaping the therapeutic encounter. The work becomes a dynamic process of co-created meaning, mutual influence, and emergent change.

In this chapter, I outline a model that integrates relational psychoanalysis, developmental science, and neurobiological research into a coherent

DOI: 10.4324/9781003789727-19

clinical framework. It is a model grounded in the realities of practice – the ruptures, repairs, enactments, and moments of unexpected aliveness that move therapy forward. It offers clinicians a way to think about the therapeutic relationship not as a technique but as a living system capable of generating new possibilities for experience.

The chapter is presented here largely as it was originally written. I have chosen not to revise it substantially, as it represents a coherent formulation that continues to inform my clinical work. If anything, subsequent developments in attachment research, relational neuroscience, and epigenetics have served to deepen and extend the questions it raises rather than render them obsolete.

Contemporary relational psychoanalysis emerged in the 1980s in the United States in an attempt to integrate interpersonal psychoanalysis with British object relations theory. A relational perspective emphasises the salience of early formative relationships on the development of personality and argues that the subject's primary motivation is to seek relationships with others. By contrast, classical Freudian thinking views motivation in terms of intrapsychic drives of sexuality and aggression. Stephen Mitchell was a prominent figure in the development of relational psychoanalysis and is widely acknowledged as the founder of the relational tradition. He established the international journal *Psychoanalytic Dialogues*, serving as its editor for the journal's first decade. Following Mitchell's untimely death in 2000, his work has been carried forward by a number of analysts and authors, including Lewis Aron, Jessica Benjamin, Philip Bromberg, Jody Davies, Emanuel Ghent, Adrienne Harris, Irwin Hoffman, Karen Maroda, Stuart Pizer, and Owen Renik.

Influenced by Fairbairn and Winnicott, Mitchell (1988) views psychopathology as characterised by constricted patterns of relatedness, with missing needs being regarded as a function of the interactive relational field. The patient's problems are seen as stemming from their tie to familiar but seriously constricted relational patterns within which the self is experienced as false, fraudulent and inauthentic. In essence, therefore, the patient must choose between remaining attached to fantasised images which impart a subtle sense of safety and connection, and the possibility of attaining attachment to real others.

For Mitchell (1988), then, the central process of treatment is the relinquishment of adaptive, defensive ties to constricted relational patterns as this will allow the patient to experience an openness to new and richer interpersonal relations. He views the affective interaction between analyst and patient as characterised by warmth and spontaneity. In this context, he stresses that the analyst must at times be prepared to take risks in order to connect with the patient in a real and authentic fashion. However, he suggests that the analyst should express their own subjectivity not only through affective interaction but also through interpretative activity. By a combination of these means, the analyst becomes a particular sort of new object to the patient, different from early parental objects. Indeed, Mitchell (1988) concludes that the analytic relationship provides the opportunity for the patient to integrate intrapsychic and interpersonal experiences in a different, more enriching and adaptive fashion than was possible in their family of origin.

The following clinical vignette is from Mitchell's book, *Relationality: From Attachment Theory to Intersubjectivity* (Mitchell, 2000). The brief vignette illustrates the founding principles of relational psychoanalysis: an integrative approach that explores the way in which early traumatic experience impacts on personality development and may create difficulties in forming and sustaining mutually rewarding and enriching relationships in later life.

Clinical Illustration

"George" is a man in his mid-20s whose wife had left him because he was "unexciting and distant". The implications of George's early sexually abusive relationship with his uncle, which apparently included oral and anal penetration, bondage and being dressed in female clothes, emerged during the course of his analysis with a female analyst. Aspects of these memories and associated dynamics were relived in the transference. This notwithstanding, George began to experiment with cross-dressing and to masturbate to sadomasochistic scenarios on the internet. He felt in the powerful grip of the traumatic memories, which he found both degrading and stimulating. The impulse to reenact the abuse continued, despite his having developed an emotionally and sexually satisfying relationship with a woman. On saying goodbye to his girlfriend after an intimate weekend together, George was plagued with what he considered to be perverse, ego-alien impulses to engage in kinky masturbatory experiences and sadomasochistic activities instead of savouring the intimate pleasures of the weekend with his girlfriend.

As Mitchell (2000) points out, there are many possible ways of understanding this sequence. He details how Fairbairn might have thought about the case material from an object relations perspective. From this approach, Mitchell (2000) suggests that George's internal object relation with his uncle

> provided some of the most intense, passionate moments of his childhood. The excitement, the sense of drama, mystery, the forbidden that characterised his uncle's experience also became George's experience. George's lustful impulses were not just vehicles to tie him *to* his uncle; they also *were* his uncle, and, through the boundary-permeable affective intensity of those moments, they were George *himself*, at his most excited, most adventurous, most alive.
>
> (Mitchell, 2000, p. 114, italics in original)

In thinking about George's adhesive, seemingly addictive, attachment to the internalised relation to the abusive uncle, Mitchell (2000) cites van der Kolk's (1994) neurobiological findings, observing that there is a physiology of attachment to early objects. Thus, George's seemingly addictive propensity repeatedly to forge interpersonal relationships redolent of ties to early objects, even when these were traumatic and ego-dystonic, may reflect neurochemical as well as psychological derivatives. In the light of van der Kolk's findings, Mitchell (2000) concludes that: "Early experiences are addictive, not just because of their psychological salience but also because of their neurochemical concomitants" (p. 115).

Liotti's (1999) motivational conceptual framework may be used to supplement Mitchell's Fairbairnian and neurobiological understanding of the depicted sequence in the context of George's early interpersonal experiences. Writing from an attachment and trauma perspective, Liotti (1999) argues that in order to avoid the painful, confusing experience of dissociation to which a contradictory, multiple self-representation developed in childhood is linked, the person may defensively inhibit the attachment motivational system by choosing, consciously or unconsciously, to activate a competing motivational system.

Liotti (1999) posits the existence of three basic motivational systems that compete with the attachment system: the agonistic, caregiving, and sexual systems. The activation of the agonistic motivational system leads the person to experience a high level of dysregulated rage and aggression, while the defensive activation of the caregiving system may lead to a form of compulsive, controlling caregiving behaviour. Alternatively, the person may choose to interact with other people on the basis of their sexual motivational system. The activation of this system creates "the basis for promiscuity and for the construction of any significant relationships according to the roles of seducer and the seduced" (p. 771).

Liotti (1999) argues that the choice of the sexual motivational system is facilitated if the person has been sexually abused by an attachment figure. He contends that the three patterns of interpersonal relationships, based on the abnormal activation of the agonistic, caregiving, and sexual motivational systems, are selected in the service of avoiding painful attachment experiences. He suggests that these sub-optimal systems may readily be observed in clinical practice in the treatment of people suffering from dissociative processes.

As Mitchell (2000) notes, "contemporary interpersonalists and theorists of intersubjectivity have contributed to our understanding of the ways in which the vicissitudes of early attachment experiences play themselves out in current relationships, including the transference-countertransference relationship with the analyst" (p. 101).

Employing an integrated model, in the context of George's early traumatic experience of sexual abuse, the separation from his girlfriend after their pleasurable weekend together may be seen as a stressful event. For patients with a traumatic history such as George's, even a relatively minor stressor may trigger a disproportionate, fearful reaction which cannot readily be terminated (Perry et al., 1995; Schore, 2001). George's excessive reaction may itself be seen as indicating that implicitly encoded traumatic memories associated with his unresolved childhood trauma had been activated, leading to a concomitant release of stress-related neurochemicals. In consequence, the secure, coherent representational model that was available to George while he was in the reassuring and comforting presence of his girlfriend was overwhelmed, and the multiple, disorganised mental model in relation to the abusing uncle was activated in a context of separation and temporary loss.

I have found that exploring with my patients in minute detail the relational context in which such shifts in representational models, object relations, or self-states occur to be a crucial aspect of the therapeutic process. Such shifts and nuances of attachment phenomena (Slade, 2004) are motivated by dissociated memories and manifested as emotional procedures in the nonverbal, implicit/enactive domain of relating and experiencing (Bruschweiler-Stern et al., 2002, 2007; Lyons-Ruth et al., 1998; Stern et al., 1998a, 1998b).

As George lacked a coherent strategy to deal with the stress of separation, the experience was dissociated or defensively excluded from consciousness. Thus, George "chose" to inhibit the attachment motivational system in order to avoid experiencing painful affect associated with his girlfriend leaving and instead activated the sexual motivational system (Liotti, 1999). Being unable to reflect upon and organise this mildly stressful attachment-related event, it would seem that George experienced it in the mode of psychic equivalence (Fonagy et al., 2002). This mode of functioning reflects the difficulty that George has in differentiating inner reality from external reality in stressful interpersonal contexts. Thus, when left alone after the pleasurable weekend with his girlfriend, George was unable to mentalise the experience and so succumbed to the impulse to seek comfort and solace in masturbatory fantasies and sadomasochistic activities with strangers on the internet as a maladaptive form of affect regulation (Schore, 1994). Moreover, as Mitchell (2000) points out, George's adhesive attachment to the internalised uncle, as manifested in repetitive reenactments of the sexual abuse, would seem to be maintained by neurochemical as well as psychological derivatives.

Given this, I would argue that George's addictive attachment is as much to a psychobiological state as to an actual person. In this sense, his relationship to the other predominantly serves as a vehicle to reexperience a familiar, albeit traumatic, state of mind. An intimate, emotionally meaningful relationship with a real other does not carry this valence for George and thus is unlikely to be sustained, as appears to have been the case in his marriage. The description of George as being "unexciting and distant" in the relationship with his wife would indicate that he had developed a dismissing state of mind in respect of attachment, and therefore employs deactivating strategies and distancing procedures to regulate his discomfort with emotional intimacy.

In terms of Ferenczi's (1933) concept of identification with the aggressor, as an abused, helpless child it is likely that George became oblivious of himself, passively gratifying the desires of his abusive uncle. In negating himself in this way, George was transformed into the image that his uncle had of him – as an object to be used and abused. Ferenczi's (1933) theory may partly account for the passive aspects of George's personality and behaviour. The more active part of George, in the form of physical and emotional withdrawal from others, may partly be understood by reference to Anna Freud's (1993) later formulation of identification with the aggressor. In this instance, George may be seen as identifying with a caregiver who routinely turned away from him, leaving him too alone.

In contrast to Ferenczi (1933), Anna Freud (1993) views identification with the aggressor as a defensive process whereby the individual transforms himself "from the person threatened into the person who makes the threat" (p. 113). For Anna Freud, the change from the passive role to the active role is a means of assimilating "dissociated" traumatic experience which is turned into "an active assault on the outside world" (p. 116). As Frankel (2002) notes, both forms of identification with the aggressor may be in operation simultaneously, being used to adapt to a threatening external reality, as well as to cope with disturbing inner feelings that arise as a result of a threat to the self.

Mitchell (2000) does not provide any details of George's developmental history, other than the sexual abuse by his uncle, as the main purpose of the vignette is to illustrate Fairbairn's thinking in respect of impulses and guilt. It may nevertheless be accepted that this traumatic experience alone set George on a developmental trajectory characterised by anxiety and insecurity, and a concomitant difficulty in sustaining an emotionally enriching intimate relationship. However, early trauma and abuse occur within an ongoing relational context. This being so, George's attachment history and the characteristic intersubjective/attachment system within which he experienced the trauma may be as salient to his personality development and adult psychopathology as the abuse itself.

In the absence of more details about the quality of George's early and current relationships with his parents, ex-wife and girlfriend, as well as his discrete discourse style in interaction with his analyst, my conjecture from an attachment perspective, as set out above, must remain just that, conjecture. While not wanting to minimise the traumatic impact on George of the sexual abuse by his uncle, I would agree with Mitchell (2000) that we need to take account of the broader developmental picture, too, in terms of cumulative relational trauma, in understanding the quality of our adult patients' intersubjective relationships.

Clinical Implications of a Developmental Perspective

Mitchell's (2000) case vignette of George illustrates the way in which implicit/procedural memory creates a bridge between early childhood experiences and psychopathology in adulthood. The case also shows how a neurobiological and developmental perspective may be integrated with a relational model in clinical work with adults. Indeed, writers such as Emde (1980), Hurry (1998), and Schore (1994) emphasise that developmental factors play a role in all analyses and are an important aspect of the therapeutic process. Moreover, that developmental work is rooted in the individual personalities of the patient and the therapist, and in their spontaneous interactions. This being so, developmental work requires the therapist to bring their own emotions and subjectivity more explicitly into the therapeutic encounter, as advocated by Mitchell (1988).

Indeed, Tähkä (1993) emphasises the therapist's legitimate experience of parent-like feelings of pleasure and pain as part of an appropriate developmental relationship with the patient. However, it needs to be acknowledged that there is a heightened countertransferential risk in developmental work of the therapist using the patient variously as a source of narcissistic gratification, to relieve guilt, to overcome feelings of helplessness, or to gratify their own infantile needs (Tähkä, 1993). Hurry (1998) stresses that these risks demand ongoing self-reflective monitoring of the countertransference.

The spontaneous features of developmental work also highlight the importance of the "fit" or "match" between patient and therapist. Indeed, Kantrowitz (1995), in her long-term follow-up study on this very issue, found that patient-analyst match was the major factor relevant to successful outcome, a point also emphasised by Maroda (2010). Developmental aspects of the therapeutic relationship may also be seen as reflecting what is often referred to as the "real relationship", as compared to the transference relationship. On discussing this clinical issue, Ogden (2004) observes that the quality of intimacy developed between therapist and patient will include feelings of camaraderie, playfulness, compassion, healthy flirtatiousness, charm, and enlivening humour. With regard to the latter, it is often overlooked that humour constitutes a shared, intersubjective experience that has significant therapeutic benefit (Lemma, 2000).

Developmental studies suggest that the capacity for intersubjectivity develops in tandem with a subjective sense of self in the preverbal domain of intersubjective relatedness (Stern, 1985), and in the context of an ongoing attachment relationship. Findings indicate that the developmental achievement of mentalisation is seriously compromised by attachment trauma. For the child who has been abused or indeed consistently negated, there may be a defensive avoidance of knowing the thoughts and feelings in the mind of the other. This is because the child, and later the adult, expects to discover therein a hostile, malevolent intent, and a reflection of the self as bad, shameful and, perhaps even worse, as not existing at all (Fonagy & Target, 1996; Fonagy et al., 2002; Fonagy 2008). In the light of these findings, understanding the adult patient's traumatic experience from a developmental perspective is, I would argue, crucial to informing the therapeutic relationship and the process of change, and to enhancing the patient's mentalising capacity and sense of self-agency (Bateman & Fonagy, 2004; Diamond & Kernberg, 2008; Holmes, 2010; Knox, 1999, 2001, 2003; Renn, 2012).

In the service of enhancing self-reflexivity and intersubjectivity, Aron (1996) advocates asking patients to describe anything that they might have observed about the therapist, and to speculate or fantasise about what the therapist might be thinking or feeling in relation to the patient. He argues that this form of openness and curiosity facilitates the patient's perception of the analyst as a separate subject. However, in acknowledging the limitations of our own self-awareness, Aron (1996) points to the risk both of imposing our subjectivity onto the patient and of presuming to know whether or not we are "validating" or "confirming" our patients' perceptions of us.

In my clinical experience, there are significant therapeutic gains to be made not only from inviting patients to think about what is in the therapist's mind, as advocated by Aron (1996), but also from encouraging them to explore and appraise what is in the minds of the people they interact with in their everyday lives. I would suggest that this constitutes a more fully systemic way of working, as described by Wachtel (2008). So often patients seem confused about what is motivating the behaviour and actions of their nearest and dearest, and use the therapist in a rather passive way to try to give meaning to the intentions of others. By engaging the patient in an active process of mentalisation, linked to an exploration and elaboration of the emotions associated with any given interpersonal context, they may be helped to shift out of habitual non- reflective modes into an intersubjective state of being-and-relating which understands and takes account of the other person's motivations and perspectives. As Aron (1996) points out, this intersubjective aspect of the therapeutic process may protect the patient from passively complying with, and submitting to, the therapist's power and authority in a way that reprises Winnicott's (1960) concept of the "false self".

Benjamin (1995), however, questions to what extent any aspect of subjectivity may be privileged as the truer, authentic part in relation to which other parts are false or inauthentic. Influenced, nevertheless, by Winnicott (1949, 1960, 1971), she amplifies Mahler et al.'s (1985) theory of separation-individuation, stressing the role that aggression plays in the development of intersubjectivity. Benjamin (1995) argues that mutual recognition and intersubjective relatedness are not inevitable aspects of infant development, but rather are developmental achievements linked to the quality of the mother-infant relationship, which may either be oppressive and controlling or facilitating and liberating.

The struggle for recognition brings forth aggression and thus separation. This fosters a symbolic space between mother and child. The mother's task is to balance the constant tension between assertion of the self and recognition of the other. Benjamin (1995) sees this developmental process as the necessary basis for non-coercive intersubjectivity.

Informed by developmental studies, she notes that relatedness is characterised not by continuous harmony, but by a continuous process of disruption and repair (Beebe & Lachmann, 1992). When the process of mutual recognition breaks down because of conflict in the mother-infant relationship, experience is organised predominantly intrapsychically rather than intersubjectively, the upshot of which is a struggle for power (Benjamin, 1995). Such unresolved developmental issues are likely to emerge in the transference/countertransference matrix.

Knowledge as an Aspect of Power

The asymmetry of power in the therapeutic relationship has been a concern of relational psychoanalysis since its inception. The paradigmatic shift from a classical model to a relational model emphasised concepts of mutual influence, discontinuity, multiplicity, and co-construction of subjective experience in clinical work. This shift changed the role of the therapist from an objective observer who is free from the patient's direct influence, and who provides interpretations from a detached, neutral perspective, to a two-person process in which mutual influence is ubiquitous and what the therapist knows is inevitably altered by their participation in the intersubjective field (Gabbard, 1996).

A relational/intersubjective perspective, then, recognises that there are two subjectivities in operation in the analytic enterprise and emphasises the way in which the therapist initiates behaviours and affects, as well as reacting to what the patient does in the therapy (Natterson, 1991). Moreover, there is no singular truth to be revealed, rather the patient's subjective experience and difficulties in living may be understood and co-constructed in a multiplicity of ways (Mitchell, 1993). However, as Aron (1996) and Benjamin (1992) point out, an awareness of the way in which our own subjectivities and theoretical orientations influence and limit such multiple possibilities merely raise new problems of power, in terms of a tension between mutuality and asymmetry, as well as thorny questions about what the analyst knows and does not know.

In discussing "knowledge as power", Benjamin (1992) cautions against idealising a stance of "not-knowing" in reaction to the old classical ideal of analytic certitude. Indeed, Winnicott (1971) contends that the therapist can hold up the patient's progress "because of genuinely not knowing" (p. 177). He argues that the patient's phenomenological experience of "primitive agonies" and concomitant "clinical fear" of a future breakdown is, in fact, the fear of a breakdown that has already happened but which has "not yet been remembered" (p. 177). He suggests that patients need to be told about this crucial aspect of their lived experience for which they have no memory.

In this context, Frankel (2006) acknowledges the reluctance in contemporary psychoanalytic circles to diagnose the patient out of fear that this kind of "knowing" may objectify the patient, thereby negating or obliterating their subjective experience. This notwithstanding, he argues that diagnosis is an idea that cannot easily be given up because people do have distinctive personality characteristics and limitations that endure over time. Moreover, he contends that no technique can eliminate the inherent power differential in the therapeutic relationship, or the therapist's unconscious use of this relationship for good or for ill.

In an attempt to overcome this dilemma and move away from a diagnostic medical model, Frankel (2002) proposes a relational model that includes the concept of diagnosis-of-the-moment: an interactive process that informs how the therapist responds moment-by-moment to the patient's changing self-states and multiple ways of organising subjective experience.

Similarly, Davies (2004) argues that in work with survivors of childhood sexual abuse, the therapist is required to make multiple shifting diagnoses in response both to the vicissitudes of the patient's self-states and to the different roles that the therapist is drawn into enacting in the transference/countertransference matrix. In this overall context, it needs to be kept in mind that powerlessness is a key feature of developmental trauma, and that dissociation in reaction to trauma walls off access to self-experience and emotional connection with others (Bromberg, 1998).

Aron (1998) eschews diagnosis, emphasising instead that what the therapist knows is partly informed by their observations of the patient's body, in terms of gesture, facial expression, and posture. This clinical stance is consonant with the recent discovery of the mirror neuron system (Gallese, 2009). Orbach (1995, 1999, 2004), too, highlights the use of the therapist's body countertranference to register and understand the patient's implicit affective states and communication of unconscious material.

From a relational perspective, it is assumed that these processes are mutual, and that the patient will change the therapist as part of a continuous process of bi-directional or mutual influence in the intersubjective field (Aron, 1996). This conceptualisation of the therapeutic process is consonant with the findings of developmental studies (Beebe & Lachmann, 1992, 2002), and challenges the view of countertransference as a static, intermittent event occurring in reaction to the patient's transference. Mutual influence, however, does not imply equal influence, in that the relationship can be mutual without being symmetrical (Aron, 1996). The therapist's struggle to understand and recover from "mistakes" and enactments without becoming defensive or inauthentic is seen as a central aspect of the therapeutic relationship, leading to mutual recognition and change (Aron, 1996; Benjamin, 1995; Frankel, 2002; Mitchell, 2000).

Again, this aspect of the therapeutic process is consonant with attachment research which shows that secure attachment is facilitated when ruptures to the parent-child attachment bond are repaired in a contingent and predictable way. It follows that the process of disruption and repair in clinical work with adults promotes a sense of felt security and thus the capacity to experience new information and relationship transformations in the implicit/enactive domain (Beebe et al., 2000; Lyons-Ruth et al., 1998).

We see, then, that relational psychoanalysis is in an ongoing process of integrating the empirical findings from attachment research and developmental studies. Mitchell (1988), however, strikes a note of caution, observing a certain tendency in developmental work to view the patient as an infantile self, encapsulated in an adult body – the so-called "child within" (Balint, 1968; Miller, 1991). He terms this tendency the "developmental tilt". Here, adult relational needs are collapsed into infantile neediness stemming from unsatisfied developmental needs. From this perspective, psychopathology is variously perceived in terms of frozen development, unresolved regressive residues from early life, or infantile fixations, and the patient is portrayed as a passive, inactive victim of a depriving environment.

This way of thinking may be seen in Balint's (1968) formulation of the "basic fault", which reflects the lack of care and nurturance available to the individual in early development. For Balint (1968), the therapeutic process should avoid conflict and facilitate a "benign regression". By contrast, Mitchell (1988) suggests that casting the analytic enterprise as regressive seriously distorts the nature of the analytic experience by collapsing relational needs into the kinds of interaction characterised by the relationship between the small child and the mother. He argues that using the metaphor of the self as baby in such a concrete, reified fashion assumes that the clinical material reflects universal infantile needs, actual memory traces, and an underlying structural dimension to the patient's experience.

Somewhat paradoxically, in his later writings Mitchell (1993) contends that in many respects the good enough caregiver-infant relationship constitutes the prototype of a therapeutic model in work with adults, and that the analytic process is redolent of the subtle intersubjective, communicative, and regulatory processes that take place between caregiver and child. His change of emphasis may reflect more recent findings in the field of attachment and developmental studies. As we have seen, these show that the internal world develops through an active, mutual process of reciprocal influence, and that the mind is composed of self-other representational models developed in the context of interaction with others.

With this integrative model in place, Chapter 15 revisits cumulative relational trauma to clarify how it functions as an organising orientation across the entire volume.

References

Aron, L. (1996). *A meeting of minds: Mutuality in psychoanalysis*. Hillsdale, NJ: Analytic Press.

Aron, L. (1998). Knowing, not-knowing and the "unknown". *Psychoanalytic Dialogues*, 8, 135–172.

Balint, M. (1968). *The basic fault: Therapeutic aspects of regression*. London: Tavistock Publications.

Bateman, A. & Fonagy, P. (2004). *Psychotherapy for borderline personality disorder: Mentalization-based treatment*. Oxford: Oxford University Press.

Beebe, B. & Lachmann, F. M. (1992). Co-constructing inner and relational processes: Self- and mutual regulation in infant research and adult treatment. *Psychoanalytic Psychology*, 9, 131–157.

Beebe, B., Lachmann, F. M. & Jaffe, J. (2000). Mother–infant interaction structures and presymbolic self and object representations. *Psychoanalytic Dialogues*, 10(2), 133–182.

Beebe, B. & Lachmann, F. M. (2002). *Infant research and adult treatment: Co-constructing interactions*. Hillsdale, NJ: Analytic Press.

Benjamin, J. (1992). *The bonds of love: Psychoanalysis, feminism, and the problem of domination*. New York: Pantheon.

Benjamin, J. (1995). *Like subjects, love objects: Essays on recognition and sexual difference*. New Haven: Yale University Press.

Bromberg, P. (1998). *Standing in the spaces: Essays on clinical process, trauma, and dissociation*. Hillsdale, NJ: Analytic Press.

Bruschweiler-Stern, N., Harrison, A. M., Lyons-Ruth, K., Morgan, A. C., Nahum, J. P., Sander, L., Stern, D. N. & Tronick, E. Z. (2002). Explicating the implicit: The local level and the microprocess of change in the analytic situation. *International Journal of Psychoanalysis*, 83(5), 1051–1062.

Bruschweiler-Stern, N., Harrison, A. M., Lyons-Ruth, K., Morgan, A. C., Nahum, J. P., Sander, L. W., Stern, D. N. & Tronick, E. Z. (2007). The process of therapeutic change involving implicit knowledge: The "something more" than interpretation. *Infant Mental Health Journal*, 28, 300–308.

Davies, J. M. (2004). Whose bad objects are we anyway? Repetition and our elusive love affair with evil. *Psychoanalytic Dialogues*, 14, 711–732.

Diamond, D. & Kernberg, O. F. (2008). Mentalization and attachment theory in the treatment of borderline personality disorder. *Journal of the American Psychoanalytic Association*, 56, 555–577.

Emde, R. (1980). Emotional availability: A reciprocal reward system for infants and parents. *Infant Mental Health Journal*, 1, 1–6.

Fairbairn, W. R. D. (1952). *Psychoanalytic studies of the personality*. London: Tavistock Publications.

Ferenczi, S. (1933). Confusion of tongues between adults and the child. *International Journal of Psychoanalysis*, 14, 225–230.

Fonagy, P. (2008). The mentalization-focused approach to social development. In F. N. Busch (ed.), *Mentalization: Theoretical considerations, research findings, and clinical implications* (pp. 3–56). Hove: Analytic Press.

Fonagy, P. & Target, M. (1996). Playing with reality: I. Theory of mind and the normal development of psychic reality. *International Journal of Psychoanalysis*, 77, 217–233.

Fonagy, P., Gergely, G., Jurist, E. & Target, M. (2002). *Affect regulation, mentalization, and the development of the self*. New York: Other Press.

Frankel, J. (2002). Exploring the sense of agency in the therapeutic relationship. *Psychoanalytic Dialogues*, 12, 171–210.

Frankel, J. (2006). The persistent sense of badness: The moral dimension of identification with the aggressor. *Psychoanalytic Quarterly*, 75, 807–844.

Freud, A. (1993). *The ego and the mechanisms of defence*. London: Karnac Books.

Gabbard, G. O. (1996). *Love and hate in the analytic setting*. Northvale, NJ: Jason Aronson.

Gallese, V. (2009). Mirror neurons, embodied simulation, and the neural basis of social identification. *Psychoanalytic Dialogues*, 19, 519–536.

Holmes, J. (2010). *Exploring in security: Towards an attachment-informed psychoanalytic psychotherapy*. London: Routledge.
Hurry, A. (1998). *Psychoanalysis and developmental therapy*. London: Karnac Books.
Kantrowitz, J. (1995). The patient's impact on the analyst. *Psychoanalytic Quarterly*, 64, 431–455.
Knox, J. (1999). The relevance of attachment theory to psychoanalysis. *British Journal of Psychotherapy*, 15, 417–432.
Knox, J. (2001). The role of mental representations in the relationship between analyst and patient. *Journal of Analytical Psychology*, 46, 613–632.
Knox, J. (2003). *Archetype, attachment, analysis: Jungian psychology and the emergent mind*. London: Routledge.
Lemma, A. (2000). *Humour in psychoanalysis*. London: Karnac Books.
Liotti, G. (1999). Disorganized attachment, dissociation and dissociative disorders. *Dissociation*, 12, 171–183.
Lyons-Ruth, K., Bronfman, E. & Parsons, E. (1998). Maternal frightened/frightening behaviour, disorganized infant attachment, and the risk for psychopathology. In J. Solomon & C. George (eds), *Attachment disorganization* (pp. 33–70). New York: Guilford Press.
Mahler, M. S., Pine, F. & Bergman, A. (1985). *The psychological birth of the human infant: Symbiosis and individuation*. London: Karnac Books.
Maroda, K. (2010). *Psychodynamic techniques: Working with emotion in the therapeutic relationship*. New York: Guilford Press.
Miller, A. (1991). *Breaking down the wall of silence: The liberating experience of facing painful truth*. New York: Dutton.
Mitchell, S. A. (1988). *Relational concepts in psychoanalysis*. Cambridge, MA: Harvard University Press.
Mitchell, S. A. (1993). *Hope and dread in psychoanalysis*. New York: Basic Books.
Mitchell, S. A. (2000). *Relationality: From attachment to intersubjectivity*. Hillsdale, NJ: Analytic Press.
Natterson, J. (1991). *The therapist's use of self*. Northvale, NJ: Jason Aronson.
Ogden, T. H. (2004). The analytic third: Implications for psychoanalytic theory and technique. *International Journal of Psychoanalysis*, 85, 1–19.
Orbach, S. (1995). *What's really going on here?* London: Penguin.
Orbach, S. (1999). *The impossibility of sex*. London: Penguin.
Orbach, S. (2004). *The body in clinical practice*. London: Routledge.
Perry, B. D., Pollard, R. A., Blakely, T. L., Baker, W. L. & Vigilante, D. (1995). Childhood trauma, the neurobiology of adaptation, and "use-dependent" development of the brain. *Infant Mental Health Journal*, 16, 271–291.
Renn, P. (2012). *The silent past and the invisible present: Memory, trauma, and representation in psychotherapy*. New York: Routledge.
Schore, A. N. (1994). *Affect regulation and the origin of the self: The neurobiology of emotional development*. Hillsdale, NJ: Lawrence Erlbaum Associates.
Schore, A. N. (2001). The effects of early relational trauma on right brain development. *Infant Mental Health Journal*, 22, 201–269.
Slade, A. (2004). Parental reflective functioning: An introduction. *Attachment & Human Development*, 6, 31–47.
Stern, D. N. (1985). *The interpersonal world of the infant*. New York: Basic Books.
Stern, D. N., Sander, L. W., Nahum, J. P., Harrison, A. M., Lyons-Ruth, K., Morgan, A. C., Bruschweiler-Stern, N. & Tronick, E. Z. (1998a). The process of therapeutic

change involving implicit knowledge: The "something more" than interpretation. *Infant Mental Health Journal*, 19, 300–308.

Stern, D. N., Sander, L. W., Nahum, J. P., Harrison, A. M., Lyons-Ruth, K., Morgan, A. C., Bruschweiler-Stern, N. & Tronick, E. Z. (1998b). Nonverbal knowing and implicit relational knowledge. *Psychoanalytic Dialogues*, 8, 843–860.

Tähkä, V. (1993). *Mind and its treatment: A psychoanalytic approach*. Madison, CT: International Universities Press.

van der Kolk, B. A. (1994). The body keeps the score. *Harvard Review of Psychiatry*, 1, 253–265.

Wachtel, P. (2008). *Relational theory and the practice of psychotherapy*. New York: Guilford Press.

Winnicott, D. W. (1949). Hate in the countertransference. *International Journal of Psychoanalysis*, 30, 69–74.

Winnicott, D. W. (1960). Ego distortion in terms of true and false self. In D. W. Winnicott, *The maturational processes and the facilitating environment* (pp. 140–152). London: Hogarth Press.

Winnicott, D. W. (1971). *Playing and reality*. London: Tavistock.

15 Cumulative Relational Trauma Revisited

Why Revisit Cumulative Relational Trauma?

Having established an integrative framework in the previous chapter, we can now revisit cumulative relational trauma. This concept has been explored in depth earlier in this volume, where it is distinguished from discrete traumatic events and situated within a developmental and relational framework. The purpose of returning to the concept here is not to extend it theoretically, but to reconsider it in light of the ground already covered. Having moved through questions of attachment, memory, dissociation, enactment, and therapeutic process, the task now is to ask how cumulative trauma appears when viewed from a wider clinical and conceptual perspective.

As argued in the preceding chapters, cumulative trauma functions less as a discrete explanatory concept than as an organising orientation towards development, suffering, and change. In this sense, it provides a language for forms of suffering that are often elusive and resistant to event-based accounts of trauma. At this point in the book, then, it can be understood as a concept that cuts across diagnostic categories and clinical presentations. Revisiting it allows us to clarify what becomes visible when development, relationship, culture, and biology are held together over time.

From Concept to Organising Orientation

Seen retrospectively, cumulative trauma describes not simply early relational adversity, but the gradual accumulation of experience across development. It draws attention away from isolated failures or dramatic ruptures and towards the ongoing texture of relational life: repeated misattunements, inconsistent recognition, and failures of repair that quietly shape expectations of self and other.

Approached in this way, difficulties often described in terms of personality, character, or chronic relational dysfunction can be understood as adaptive responses to environments in which recognition, containment, or influence were repeatedly compromised. What later appears as rigidity,

DOI: 10.4324/9781003789727-20

withdrawal, or volatility may reflect efforts to preserve coherence in the absence of reliable relational regulation. Cumulative trauma thus provides a way of thinking about continuity without linear causality, and about development without assuming either inevitability or deficit. It allows clinicians to remain attentive to history without becoming captive to it.

Influence, Agency, and the Experience of Powerlessness

One aspect of cumulative trauma that comes into sharper focus when revisited concerns the child's experience of influence within early relationships. Beyond misattunement lies a more corrosive experience: that one's signals fail to register, that one's distress does not alter the relational field, and that one's presence makes little difference to those on whom one depends.

Over time, this experience may shape a deep sense of powerlessness. In some individuals, this is expressed through compliance, emotional inhibition, or a reluctance to make claims on others; in others, through protest, aggression, or controlling strategies aimed at forcing recognition. In both cases, the underlying issue is not simply unmet need, but the repeated failure of action to have effect.

Clinically, this dimension of cumulative trauma is often encountered in the therapeutic relationship, where patients test – sometimes quietly, sometimes forcefully – whether their communications will be received and whether their experience can influence the other. These expectations are held implicitly, shaping relational engagement long before they can be reflected upon.

Cultural, Systemic, and Intergenerational Contexts

Revisiting cumulative trauma also brings its cultural and systemic dimensions into clearer view. Early relational environments are embedded within broader social and historical contexts that shape caregivers' capacities for attunement, regulation, and availability. Chronic stressors such as poverty, racism, displacement, and social marginalisation exert pressure on relational systems, increasing the likelihood of cumulative relational strain without implying individual failure or intent.

From an intergenerational perspective, cumulative trauma is often transmitted through patterns of regulation and expectation rather than through explicit narrative. Caregivers shaped by their own histories of deprivation or dislocation may struggle to offer forms of recognition and repair that were absent in their own development. In this way, cumulative trauma is carried not only within individuals, but within families, communities, and social structures, as discussed in Chapter 8. Holding these dimensions together allows clinicians to resist reductive explanations. It situates cumulative trauma within a matrix of relational, cultural, and structural forces, supporting a stance of compassion without blame and responsibility without moralism.

Clinical Implications: Working with What Has Accumulated

Adopting a cumulative perspective brings subtle but important shifts in clinical practice. Assessment moves away from the search for discrete traumatic events and towards attention to patterns: how affect is regulated, how influence is negotiated, and how expectations of recognition emerge in the therapeutic relationship. These subtle aspects of the clinical encounter can be seen in my work with Patricia in Chapter 9, and with Katarina in Chapter 11.

Therapeutic action similarly shifts emphasis. Because cumulative trauma is encoded implicitly and procedurally, change rarely occurs through insight alone. Instead, it depends on repeated experiences of attunement, reliability, and repair, through which new expectations can gradually take root. The therapeutic relationship becomes a site where influence can be restored, signals can be received, and agency tentatively re-experienced. This way of working demands patience and a tolerance for slow change. Yet it also opens the possibility of profound transformation, as patterns that once felt fixed begin to soften and reorganise.

Limits, Tensions, and Open Questions

Revisiting cumulative trauma also requires acknowledging its limits. As a concept, it risks overextension if applied indiscriminately, or treated as a totalising explanation. It is best held as an orienting framework rather than a comprehensive theory – valuable precisely because it invites complexity rather than closure.

Questions remain regarding its relationship to diagnostic systems, its interface with neurodevelopmental conditions, and its place within increasingly biomedical models of mental health. Rather than resolving these tensions, cumulative trauma brings them into focus, underscoring the importance of holding multiple explanatory perspectives in dialogue. In this sense, cumulative trauma remains less a settled construct than an ongoing clinical orientation – one that invites clinicians to listen for what has accumulated silently over time, and to remain attentive to the relational conditions under which change becomes possible.

Transition to Chapter 16

In sum, revisiting cumulative trauma reveals that it is not a discrete category but rather an orienting framework – one that illuminates how suffering becomes organised over time and how therapeutic change depends on sustained relational experience rather than singular insight. Revisiting cumulative trauma in this way prepares the ground for a final consideration of how contemporary neuroscience might be thought about, rather than relied upon, in relational clinical practice. The question that follows is not what neuroscience can explain, but how it can be integrated without eclipsing the relational, developmental, and cultural dimensions that remain central to therapeutic work – how it can be held within a relational-developmental framework while preserving the experiential and interpersonal dimensions of clinical work.

16 Integrative Reflections on Relational Neuroscience

Why Neuroscience Invites Reflection Rather than Accumulation

Chapter 14 has shown how neuroscience can be productively integrated with attachment and psychoanalytic thinking. The question, then, is not *whether* to incorporate it, but *how* to hold it.

Over the past two decades, neuroscience has come to occupy an increasingly prominent place within psychoanalytic and psychotherapeutic discourse. Findings from affective neuroscience, developmental neurobiology, and trauma research have offered compelling accounts of regulation, memory, and plasticity, often lending empirical support to clinical observations long familiar to psychoanalytic practitioners. At the same time, the rapid uptake of neuroscientific language has raised questions about how such knowledge should be integrated into clinical thinking without eclipsing the relational and experiential foundations of therapeutic work.

The purpose of this chapter is not to review neuroscientific findings, nor to extend the range of concepts already discussed elsewhere in this volume. Rather, it is to reflect on the *status* of neuroscience within relational clinical practice: what it offers, where its limits lie, and how it can be thought about productively without becoming explanatory or prescriptive. In this sense, the chapter is concerned less with neuroscience as a body of knowledge than with how clinicians make use of it in thinking about change.

What Neuroscience Genuinely Contributes to Relational Practice

Neuroscience has made valuable contributions to clinical understanding, particularly in relation to affect regulation, implicit memory, and the embodied nature of experience. Concepts such as co-regulation, stress-response systems, and neural plasticity have provided clinicians with a language for articulating processes that were previously described only metaphorically or inferred indirectly through clinical observation.

Within a relational framework, these contributions are most useful when they illuminate *process* rather than explain outcome. Neurobiological research has helped clarify how early relational experiences shape regulatory capacities, how repeated patterns of interaction become embedded procedurally, and how new experiences can gradually modify these patterns

DOI: 10.4324/9781003789727-21

over time. In this respect, neuroscience has supported a shift away from insight-based models of change towards a greater appreciation of repetition, reliability, and affective engagement.

Importantly, these findings do not introduce new clinical aims so much as they deepen our understanding of familiar ones. They lend coherence to long-standing clinical intuitions regarding the importance of presence, timing, and repair, and help clinicians tolerate the slowness with which meaningful change often unfolds.

The Risks of Privileging Neuroscience

At the same time, the growing authority of neuroscience carries risks when it is granted explanatory primacy. One such risk is a drift towards biological determinism, in which complex relational phenomena are reduced to brain states or neurochemical processes. Another is the temptation to seek technical solutions to problems that are fundamentally relational, ethical, or developmental in nature.

When neuroscience is over-privileged, it can obscure questions of meaning, agency, and context. It may encourage clinicians to locate difficulty within the individual organism rather than within relational systems, or to conceptualise suffering in ways that detach it from lived experience. In these instances, neuroscience risks becoming a language of closure rather than curiosity.

From a relational perspective, this is particularly problematic. The therapeutic relationship cannot be reduced to mechanisms of regulation or neural synchrony without losing its ethical and experiential dimensions. While neurobiological accounts may describe *how* change becomes possible, they cannot determine *what* change means, nor can they replace the clinical task of engaging with the patient's subjective world.

Holding Neuroscience Relationally

The challenge, then, is not whether to incorporate neuroscience, but *how* to hold or contain it. Within a relational clinical stance, neuroscience is most useful when treated as one level of description among others – complementary rather than authoritative. It can inform clinical thinking without dictating it, offering metaphors and frameworks that support reflection rather than foreclose it.

Held relationally, neuroscience encourages clinicians to remain attentive to process: to moments of attunement and misattunement, to shifts in affective tone, and to the ways in which experience is regulated within relationship. It supports a view of change as emergent and progressive, grounded in repeated relational experiences rather than dramatic insight or technical intervention.

This stance also requires epistemic humility. Neuroscientific findings are provisional, evolving, and context-dependent, and they gain clinical meaning only when translated into lived relational experience. Recognising this allows clinicians to draw on neuroscience without becoming beholden to it.

Neuroscience, Cumulative Relational Trauma, and the Limits of Explanation

When considered alongside cumulative relational trauma, the limits of neuroscientific explanation become particularly evident. While neuroscience can describe the effects of chronic stress on regulatory systems, it cannot fully account for the relational meanings of such experience, nor for the ways in which power, influence, and recognition shape development over time.

Cumulative trauma, as explored throughout this volume, highlights the importance of relational context and agency. Its repair depends not only on changes in regulation but on the restoration of influence within relationship – the experience of being able to affect another and to be held in mind. These dimensions cannot be reduced to neural processes, even though they may be supported by them. In this sense, neuroscience can accompany but not substitute for a relational understanding of trauma. It can help clinicians remain patient and grounded in the face of slow change, but it cannot resolve the ethical and interpersonal questions that remain central to therapeutic work.

An Integrative Stance Moving Forward

An integrative relational practice does not require allegiance to neuroscience nor resistance to it. What it requires is the capacity to hold multiple perspectives in dialogue, recognising that each illuminates different aspects of the same complex phenomena. Neuroscience, attachment theory, and psychoanalysis each offer partial views, and their integration depends less on synthesis than on ongoing conversation.

For clinicians, this means remaining oriented towards relationship, meaning, and experience, while drawing selectively on neuroscientific insights where they genuinely support clinical understanding. It involves resisting the allure of certainty and technical mastery, and tolerating the uncertainty inherent in working with deeply embedded relational patterns.

In this way, neuroscience becomes a companion to relational thinking rather than its destination. It offers support for a clinical stance that values patience, responsiveness, and humility – qualities that remain as essential to therapeutic work now as they were before the advent of contemporary neuroscience.

Transition to the Conclusion

The concluding chapter draws these strands together, articulating the stance required for a relational-neurodevelopmental clinical practice grounded in informed uncertainty, relational presence, and developmental understanding. The task is not to resolve complexity but to consider how it can be lived with in the ongoing encounter between therapist and patient.

17 Conclusion

Towards a Relational-Neurodevelopmental Clinical Practice

In the Introduction to this volume, I posed a question that has organised thirty years of clinical work and theoretical inquiry: *How do early relational experiences become woven into the fabric of who we are, shaping not only our own lives but also the lives of the next generation?* The chapters that precede this conclusion have approached that question from multiple vantage points – developmental, psychoanalytic, neurobiological, relational, and clinical. What has emerged is not a single answer, but a framework for thinking about development, trauma, and therapeutic change that is capable of holding complexity without being paralysed by it.

This concluding chapter draws together the central threads of the volume and reflects on their implications for clinical practice, training, and future theoretical development. It is also, inevitably, a more personal reflection on what three decades of engagement with these questions has taught me about the possibilities and limits of our work, and about the stance required to practise with integrity in the face of irreducible complexity.

Cumulative Trauma: What We Now Understand

The organising concept of this volume – cumulative trauma – has evolved considerably since Masud Khan's original formulation. What has emerged through dialogue with attachment research, infant studies, and neuroscience is a more precise understanding of how chronic relational disruption shapes development.

Cumulative trauma is now best understood as a disorder of regulation: affective, autonomic, and relational. When early caregiving repeatedly fails to provide adequate co-regulation, the developing child adapts through strategies that may preserve survival but exact long-term costs – hypervigilance, emotional constriction or flooding, dissociation, and rigid defensive organisation. These adaptations are encoded procedurally rather than narratively, carried in bodily states, patterns of expectation, and modes of relating that operate largely outside conscious awareness.

Because these adaptations shape the caregiver's later regulatory capacities, cumulative trauma is readily transmitted across generations. The

DOI: 10.4324/9781003789727-22

research reviewed throughout this volume illuminates the mechanisms through which this occurs – attachment patterns, discourse styles, epigenetic processes, stress-response systems, and embodied affective communication – providing empirical grounding for what clinicians have long observed in practice.

Perhaps most importantly, this framework allows us to recognise a form of trauma that is pervasive yet frequently overlooked precisely because it lacks dramatic rupture. Chronic misattunement, emotional absence, frightened or frightening caregiving, and failures of repair are not exceptional clinical phenomena; they are the ordinary terrain of much therapeutic work. Understanding cumulative trauma makes sense of presentations that otherwise appear puzzling or resistant and offers a non-pathologising framework for understanding suffering rooted in relational history.

Integration without Reduction

A central challenge of this book has been integration without reduction – holding multiple levels of analysis together without collapsing one into another. Several lessons emerge from this sustained effort.

First, mechanism is not meaning. Neuroscience illuminates regulatory processes and correlates of attachment and change, but it does not replace psychological or relational understanding. Human experience operates simultaneously at biological, relational, psychological, and cultural levels; adequate clinical thinking requires conceptual tools appropriate to each.

Second, biology is not destiny. Epigenetic and neurodevelopmental research demonstrates the profound impact of experience on biological systems, while also underscoring plasticity across the lifespan. Vulnerability shapes possibility but does not fix outcome.

Third, universal processes take culturally specific forms. Attachment, regulation, and development unfold within cultural and social contexts that shape meaning, expectation, and expression. Clinical work must attend carefully to culture and context without collapsing suffering into difference or ignoring the biological consequences of systemic oppression.

Fourth, systemic forces operate through bodies. Racism, poverty, migration, and marginalisation are not merely social stressors but conditions with neurobiological consequences that shape caregiving, regulation, and development. Recognising this allows us to move beyond individualised blame toward ethically grounded, context-sensitive clinical work.

Finally, integration requires humility. Despite advances across disciplines, much remains unknown. Neuroscience often raises as many questions as it answers; clinical change remains difficult to predict. A stance of informed uncertainty is therefore not a weakness, but a professional necessity.

The Therapeutic Relationship Reconsidered

If cumulative trauma is encoded procedurally and transmitted through enacted patterns of relating, then therapeutic change must occur through new relational experience, not insight alone. This places the therapeutic relationship at the centre of clinical work in a very specific way.

Throughout this volume, I have argued that the therapeutic relationship is not merely the context for technique, but the primary site of procedural transformation. The therapist's affective presence – the capacity to be genuinely engaged, moved, and responsive – matters profoundly for patients whose early experience was characterised by chronic misattunement or emotional absence. Such presence cannot be performed; it requires authenticity, regulation, and the capacity to be affected.

From this perspective, enactments are inevitable and potentially transformative. Rather than representing technical failure, they reveal implicit relational expectations seeking recognition. When enactments are recognised, acknowledged, and repaired, they offer new procedural experience: that ruptures can be named, responsibility can be shared, and connection can be restored.

Because procedural change occurs through repetition, transformation is necessarily gradual. Extended relational engagement is often required for patients whose difficulties reflect cumulative trauma. This is not a rejection of brief or structured interventions, but recognition that certain forms of developmental disruption require time, repetition, and sustained relational presence.

Implications for Training and Supervision

If therapeutic work operates significantly at the procedural level, training must address these dimensions directly. Intellectual knowledge alone is insufficient. Effective training requires experiential and relational components: personal therapy, supervision that attends to affective and relational processes, and opportunities to observe and reflect on lived clinical work.

Supervision, in particular, must engage implicit processes and enactments, providing space to reflect on the therapist's own responses without shame or defensiveness. This requires supervisors capable of working relationally and trainees supported to tolerate vulnerability and uncertainty.

Training must also engage systemic and cultural dimensions as intrinsic to clinical work. Understanding cumulative trauma requires attention to power, privilege, and social location – not as adjuncts to technique, but as central clinical concerns.

Holding Complexity: A Personal Reflection

Over time, my confidence in single explanatory systems has diminished, even as my commitment to integration has deepened. Human development is shaped by biology, relationship, culture, chance, and agency, interacting in ways we only partially understand. Early experience matters profoundly, yet later relationships can transform what once seemed fixed.

The challenge is to hold this complexity without retreating into either oversimplification or paralysis. This requires what I have come to think of as informed uncertainty – a stance that combines rigorous knowledge with humility, expertise with openness, and authority with curiosity.

Patients do not require certainty from us, but they do require presence, commitment, and the capacity to think and feel with them. Acknowledging uncertainty need not undermine therapeutic authority; it may in fact strengthen trust.

Hope and Future Possibility

Working with cumulative trauma can feel discouraging. The weight of early experience, intergenerational transmission, and systemic oppression can appear overwhelming. Yet decades of clinical work have convinced me that transformation remains possible – rarely complete, often partial, but profoundly meaningful.

Patients can develop earned security. Parents can interrupt intergenerational transmission. Relationships can become less rigid, more reflective, more alive. These changes are incremental, fragile, and never absolute – but they matter enormously.

Hope, in this framework, is grounded not in optimism but in plasticity: neural, relational, and psychological. It is grounded in the capacity for repair, in the persistence of relational influence across the lifespan, and in the fact that new experience – when sustained – can reorganise even deeply entrenched patterns.

Final Reflections

This volume has traced the pathways through which early relational experience shapes development, personality, and intergenerational transmission. It has proposed cumulative trauma as a unifying framework for understanding these processes and has situated the therapeutic relationship as the primary site where procedural transformation becomes possible.

Psychotherapy, understood in this way, is slow, demanding work. It requires tolerance for uncertainty, willingness to be affected, and sustained attention to our own development as clinicians. It calls for integration without reduction and for ethical engagement with complexity.

Above all, it requires hope grounded in realism: not that the past can be undone, but that new relational experience can open different futures. The chapters of this volume represent one practitioner's effort to understand these processes and their clinical implications. They are offered in the hope that others engaged in similar work may find here conceptual resources, clinical understanding, and a framework for thinking that supports their essential task. At the age of eighty-one, and still practising, I can confirm that the conversation continues.

Coda

We begin life in relationship, and we continue to be shaped by the relationships we develop over the course of our lives, long after childhood has passed. What this volume has sought to show is not simply how early experience leaves its mark, but how those marks can be encountered, understood, and, in part, transformed through new relational experience. The work of psychotherapy does not erase history – it offers the possibility that history need not have the final word.

Glossary

The glossary serves as an orienting companion to the volume, offering readers clear, relationally attuned definitions of the key concepts that shape a relational–neurodevelopmental approach to psychotherapy. Drawing together ideas from attachment theory, relational psychoanalysis, and contemporary neuroscience, it introduces terms in language that is clinically grounded, accessible, and sensitive to the lived experience of development.

Tracing themes from early affect regulation and co-regulation through cumulative relational trauma, mentalisation, and therapeutic transformation, the glossary mirrors the book's developmental arc. Entries highlight how neurobiological processes unfold within human relationships, and how early relational patterns continue to shape adult intimacy, resilience, and the possibilities for change within the therapeutic relationship.

More than a reference tool, the glossary supports readers in navigating the book's interdisciplinary landscape, offering conceptual clarity while reinforcing the integrative threads that run throughout the volume.

Adult attachment interview (AAI)	A semi-structured interview assessing adults' state of mind with respect to attachment by exploring their childhood experiences and current representations of those experiences. Classifications include secure-autonomous, dismissing, preoccupied, and unresolved, each of which predicts patterns of attachment in their own children.
Affect integration	The developmental process through which emotional experience becomes differentiated, tolerable, and symbolically representable within a relational context. Affect integration links bodily arousal, subjective feeling, and meaning, enabling experience to be reflected upon rather than enacted. It emerges through repeated experiences of attuned co-regulation and is often disrupted in cumulative relational trauma, leaving affective states either overwhelming or unformulated. In psychotherapy, affect integration is supported through the therapist's regulated presence, marked mirroring, and capacity to scaffold reflective meaning-making.
Affect regulation	The capacity to manage and modulate emotional states, particularly the intensity and duration of feelings. Develops through early caregiver–infant interactions and remains central to psychological wellbeing throughout life.
Affective attunement	The caregiver's capacity to match not just the content but the affective quality, intensity, and rhythm of the infant's emotional state. Stern distinguished affective attunement from simple imitation, emphasising its role in communicating shared feeling states and supporting the development of intersubjective awareness.

Affective rupture	A disruption in emotional attunement or relational continuity, experienced as misrecognition, withdrawal, mismatch, or a break in the felt sense of connection. Ruptures are inevitable in development and in therapy; their significance lies not in their occurrence but in the quality and timeliness of repair. When ruptures remain unaddressed or chronically unresolved, they contribute to cumulative relational trauma and shape procedural expectations of non-influence, rejection, or danger. Effective repair restores connection and fosters resilience, trust, and the capacity for relational flexibility.
Ambivalent-resistant attachment (anxious-ambivalent)	An insecure attachment pattern in which the infant shows heightened distress during separation, difficulty being soothed upon reunion, and conflicted behaviour towards the caregiver (approaching while also showing anger or resistance).
Amygdala	A limbic-system structure centrally involved in detecting threat, generating rapid affective responses, and encoding implicit emotional memory. The amygdala appraises environmental cues for safety or danger before conscious awareness, shaping autonomic arousal, vigilance, and defensive mobilisation. Early caregiving relationships strongly influence amygdala reactivity; consistent co-regulation supports calibrated threat detection, whereas frightening, inconsistent, or emotionally absent caregiving heightens amygdala sensitivity and contributes to the implicit fear conditioning characteristic of cumulative relational trauma. In such contexts, the amygdala becomes primed to anticipate danger even in benign relational situations, shaping hyperarousal, procedural expectations of threat, and the rapid activation of survival-based self-states. In therapeutic work, amygdala-driven shifts in affect or bodily activation often signal the emergence of traumatised relational templates that can be regulated and reorganised within an attuned, stable dyad.

Archaic representational model	Early-formed, implicitly encoded patterns of self-other relating that develop in infancy and early childhood. These models operate outside conscious awareness and may be activated during stress or in relationships that evoke attachment dynamics. Also termed "internal working models" in attachment theory.
Attachment behavioural system	An innate motivational system that promotes proximity-seeking to caregivers when the child experiences threat or distress, thereby ensuring protection and survival.
Attunement	The caregiver's capacity to recognise, respond to, and reflect the infant's emotional states in a timely, contingent, and emotionally matched manner. Repeated experiences of attunement support the development of affect regulation and secure attachment.
Avoidant attachment	An insecure attachment pattern characterised by the infant's apparent indifference to the caregiver's departure and avoidance of contact upon reunion. Although behaviourally minimising distress, avoidant infants typically show elevated physiological arousal. This pattern develops in response to consistent parental rejection or emotional unavailability.
Basal ganglia	A group of subcortical structures involved in movement regulation, habit formation, and procedural learning. The basal ganglia help automate behavioural and affective responses, linking action tendencies with implicit relational memory. Early caregiving shapes these procedural patterns; consistent co-regulation supports flexible behavioural organisation, whereas cumulative relational trauma can consolidate rigid, survival-based habits that re-emerge in therapy as familiar enactments. Within an attuned therapeutic relationship, new experiences of co-regulation can gradually modify procedural tendencies mediated by the basal ganglia, thereby increasing relational flexibility.

Congruence/contingency	In attachment research, contingency refers to the temporal relationship between infant signal and caregiver response (how quickly and reliably caregivers respond). Congruence refers to the qualitative match between infant state and caregiver response (emotional appropriateness). Both are essential for secure attachment development.
Containment	The process by which one person receives, processes, and transforms another's unmanageable emotional experience into a form that can be tolerated and re-internalised. Containment involves the capacity to hold affect without becoming overwhelmed or retaliatory, offering it back in a metabolised, thinkable form. In development, containment enables the child to recognise, regulate, and symbolise emotional states. In cumulative relational trauma, failures of containment leave affect unprocessed or dissociated. Within psychotherapy, containment supports the integration of previously unmentalised experience and fosters the emergence of reflective capacity.
Contingent responsivity	The caregiver's ability to respond predictably and appropriately to the infant's signals and communications, fostering a sense of agency and relational expectation in the child.
Co-regulation	The process by which a caregiver helps regulate the infant's emotional and physiological states through attuned, responsive interaction. Co-regulation provides the scaffolding from which self-regulation gradually develops. When inconsistent or absent, the child may rely on maladaptive autonomic strategies that contribute to cumulative trauma.

Countertransference	The therapist's emotional, bodily, and relational responses to the patient, shaped by both the therapist's own history and the patient's enacted relational templates. In contemporary relational theory, countertransference is understood as an inevitable, co-constructed phenomenon and a primary source of information about the patient's implicit relational knowing. Countertransference responses often signal emerging enactments, dissociated self-states, or "now moments" within the dyad and can facilitate procedural transformation when recognised and worked with reflectively.
Cumulative relational trauma	The developmental impact of repeated relational disruptions – such as misattunement, inconsistent caregiving, and unresolved affective ruptures – that occur in the absence of discrete traumatic events. Cumulative trauma is encoded in implicit memory and transmitted intergenerationally through procedural patterns of relating. Impacts the capacity to develop trust, regulate affect within relationships, and develop secure attachment. Chronic failures of repair are central to its formation.
Cybernetics (in attachment theory)	A framework concerned with regulation, control, and communication in systems through feedback processes. Bowlby incorporated cybernetic principles to describe the attachment behavioural system as goal-corrected and feedback-regulated, continuously monitoring and adjusting proximity to caregivers in response to perceived threat and internal state. Cybernetics specifies the regulatory mechanisms through which attachment behaviour is dynamically organised and adapted in context.
Developmental organisation	The patterned structuring of affect regulation, relational expectation, and defensive strategy that emerges over time through repeated experience. In cumulative relational trauma, disturbance lies less in isolated events than in the organisation of the self-in-relation across development.

Developmental tilt (Mitchell)	Stephen Mitchell's early critique of psychoanalysis highlighted a "developmental tilt" – the field's tendency to privilege early childhood as the primary organiser of adult relational life. He initially emphasised the ongoing, co-constructed nature of adult relationships, cautioning against over-locating meaning in infancy. In later work, informed by infant research and attachment theory, Mitchell revised this position, acknowledging the formative weight of early asymmetrical caregiving and its enduring influence on implicit relational patterns. His shift reflects the broader integration of developmental science within relational theory.
Discourse coherence	In attachment research, the manner in which narratives about relationships are constructed and communicated. Discourse coherence – characterised by collaborative engagement, narrative clarity, and balanced consideration of experience – is associated with secure attachment. Discourse patterns (e.g., dismissive minimisation, preoccupied entanglement, or unresolved lapses) reveal implicit relational expectations and procedural strategies.
Disorganised/disoriented attachment	An attachment pattern marked by contradictory, incomplete, or disoriented behaviours during reunion with the caregiver (e.g., approaching with head averted, freezing). Most strongly associated with frightening or frightened caregiving and unresolved parental trauma.
Dissociation	An alteration in consciousness in which aspects of experience are split off from awareness, often occurring when psychological defences are overwhelmed. Dissociation exists on a continuum and, in trauma, may result in memories being fragmented into sensory or affective elements without narrative coherence.
DNA methylation	An epigenetic mechanism in which methyl groups attach to DNA, modulating gene expression without altering the genetic code itself. One pathway through which early relational experience, stress, and broader social conditions influence neurobiological functioning and can be transmitted across generations.

Earned secure attachment	A classification describing adults whose current attachment state of mind is secure-autonomous despite histories of insecure or traumatic childhood attachment. Typically achieved through sustained reflective processes, psychotherapy, or significant corrective relational experiences.
Ego-dystonic	Experiences, impulses, or self-states that feel alien, conflictual, or inconsistent with one's sense of self. Ego-dystonic material often reflects dissociated affect, unmentalised experience, or relational patterns that have not yet been symbolically integrated. In therapeutic work, ego-dystonic elements frequently emerge through enactment or bodily communication and become available for integration when held within a regulated, reflective relational field.
Ego-syntonic	Experiences, behaviours, or relational patterns that feel consistent with one's sense of self and therefore are not experienced as problematic. Ego-syntonic phenomena often reflect deeply encoded procedural expectations and early relational templates that have become organised into the self--structure. Because they feel familiar and coherent, ego-syntonic patterns may persist even when they limit relational flexibility or contribute to cumulative trauma.
Embodied simulation	A process by which observing another person's actions, emotions, or sensations activates corresponding neural patterns in the observer, as if experiencing them firsthand. Thought to underlie empathy and emotional understanding.
Enactment	The behavioural expression of unconscious relational patterns, typically involving both patient and therapist in a co-created dynamic that reflects implicit procedural expectations. In contemporary relational thinking, enactments are understood as inevitable and potentially informative rather than as technical failures. Enactments are the lived expression of implicit relational memory systems within the intersubjective field.

Epigenetic plasticity	The capacity for gene expression to be dynamically shaped through reversible biochemical processes in ways that reflect developmental, environmental, and relational conditions, illustrating how lived interpersonal experience can influence biological regulation without altering the DNA sequence.
Epigenetics	The study of how environmental factors, including relational experiences and chronic stress, influence gene expression without altering the DNA sequence itself. Such changes can affect stress-response systems and may be transmitted across generations.
Epistemic trust	The capacity to regard knowledge communicated by others as trustworthy, generalisable, and relevant to oneself. Develops within secure attachment relationships when caregivers reliably demonstrate themselves as trustworthy sources of information. Fonagy and colleagues propose that cumulative trauma can create "epistemic petrification" – a defensive closure to new information that limits the capacity to benefit from therapeutic and social learning.
Erotic transference/erotic countertransference	The emergence of erotic feeling within the therapeutic relationship, understood within a relational-attachment frame not primarily as sexual impulse but as an expression of longing, recognition, and unmet developmental need. Erotic material often conveys implicit relational knowledge about intimacy, visibility, and the organisation of desire and danger within early attachment relationships. Erotic countertransference – the therapist's own erotic responsiveness – is viewed as an inevitable aspect of the intersubjective field, offering information about the patient's enacted relational templates. Its clinical value depends on the therapist's capacity to hold such experience reflectively, without enactment or defensive foreclosure, while maintaining the ethical frame and relational asymmetry that safeguard the work.

Ethology (in attachment theory)	The study of animal behaviour in natural contexts, emphasising evolutionary function and adaptive value. Bowlby drew on ethology, particularly the work of Konrad Lorenz, Harry Harlow, and Nikolaas Tinbergen, to conceptualise attachment as an innate, biologically organised behavioural system shaped by evolutionary pressures to maintain proximity to caregivers. Attachment behaviours, for example, crying, clinging, following, smiling, are understood as adaptive responses to threat, forming the evolutionary foundation of early relational organisation.
Explicit memory	Conscious, declarative memory for events and facts that can be deliberately recalled and verbally described. Develops after approximately age two to three and involves hippocampal functioning.
Frightening/frightened caregiving	Parental behaviour that is either directly frightening to the child (e.g., hostile or threatening) or marked by fearfulness in the parent's own demeanour (e.g., anxious, dissociated). Associated with disorganised infant attachment and unresolved parental trauma.

Hippocampus	A brain structure centrally involved in the consolidation of explicit, autobiographical memory and in contextualising experience in time and space. Chronic stress and trauma are associated with alterations in hippocampal functioning, contributing to fragmented or poorly integrated memory. Early caregiving relationships strongly shape hippocampal development; consistent co-regulation and reliable repair support the neural integration of affect, context, and narrative. In cumulative relational trauma – marked by chronic misattunement, non-influence, or frightening caregiving – prolonged stress activation can disrupt hippocampal maturation, leaving emotional experience encoded without temporal or narrative anchoring. This vulnerability increases the likelihood that amygdala-driven, survival-based responses will dominate, as past relational threat is experienced as occurring in the present. In psychotherapy, the therapist's regulated presence and capacity to scaffold reflective meaning-making help re-engage hippocampal processes, supporting the gradual weaving of dissociated fragments into a more coherent and temporally organised sense of self.
Holding	The caregiver's capacity to provide a reliable emotional and relational environment in which experience can be safely felt, organised, and integrated. Holding includes both physical and psychological dimensions – protection from overwhelming stimulation, consistent responsiveness, and a stable relational frame. Adequate holding supports the development of self-cohesion and affect regulation. When holding is absent or inconsistent, the child may experience impingement, fragmentation, or premature self-reliance. In therapy, holding is enacted through presence, attunement, and the maintenance of relational asymmetry.

Hyperactivation/deactivation (of attachment system)	Contrasting strategies for managing attachment needs under stress. Hyperactivation (associated with anxious/preoccupied patterns) involves intensified proximity-seeking, heightened vigilance to rejection, and difficulty being soothed. Deactivation (associated with avoidant patterns) involves minimising attachment needs, emotional suppression, and self-reliance. Both represent adaptations to inconsistent or rejecting caregiving.
Hyper-arousal/hypo-arousal	States of autonomic dysregulation reflecting extremes of the stress-response system. Hyperarousal involves heightened sympathetic activation (fight/flight), manifesting as agitation, vigilance, emotional flooding, or impulsivity. Hypo-arousal involves parasympathetic shutdown (freeze/collapse), manifesting as numbness, withdrawal, or dissociation. Cumulative trauma often leads to oscillation between these states when co-regulation and repair are insufficient.
Identification with the aggressor	A defensive adaptation in which the child internalises aspects of a threatening, unavailable, or abusive caregiver in order to maintain attachment and manage uncontained anxiety. Understood here as a relationally evoked response rather than an instinctual drive.
Implicit memory	Nonconscious memory for procedures, habits, emotional responses, and relational patterns. Predominant in early life prior to the development of explicit memory systems and continues to shape expectations, feelings, and behaviours across the lifespan.
Implicit relational knowing (IRK)	A term used by Daniel Stern and the Boston Change Process Study Group to describe non-verbal, procedurally encoded knowledge about relationships, acquired through lived experience and enacted in patterns of interaction rather than held as conscious or narrative memory.

Implicit-explicit integration	The process by which nonconscious, procedural, and affective forms of knowing become linked with conscious, symbolic, and narrative representation. This integration supports reflective functioning, temporal continuity, and a coherent sense of self. It depends on relational safety and the availability of a regulated other who can help bridge bodily experience with meaning. Trauma disrupts implicit-explicit integration, leaving experience fragmented, uncontextualised, or enacted. Therapeutically, integration occurs through co-regulation, mentalisation, and the gradual weaving of implicit relational knowing into explicit understanding.
Informed uncertainty	A disciplined clinical stance in which the therapist contains complex theoretical and neurobiological knowledge while remaining open to the unpredictable emergence of the intersubjective "now moments". It shifts the work from technical mastery to disciplined intuition, allowing the therapist to be impacted by the patient's procedural world without premature closure.
Interactionism	A perspective emphasising that psychological experience emerges within ongoing, reciprocal patterns of influence between individuals. In a relational-developmental frame, interactionism underscores that neither subjectivity nor observation can be understood in isolation; both arise within the co-created relational field. The therapist's perceptions and responses are therefore part of the system being observed, not external to it.
Intergenerational transmission	The processes by which attachment patterns, trauma, and relational expectations are passed from one generation to the next through implicit, procedural interactions rather than explicit communication.
Internal working models (IWMs)	Mental representations of the self, attachment figures, and relationships that develop from early attachment experiences. Internal working models guide expectations, behaviours, and emotional responses in relationships, largely outside conscious awareness. Also referred to as "representational models" in psychoanalytic literature.

Interpersonal neurobiology (IPNB)	A multidisciplinary framework developed by Daniel Siegel that views the mind as an emergent, self-organising process shaped by the continuous interaction of brain, body, and relationships. IPNB identifies integration – the linking of differentiated neural and relational processes – as the core mechanism of psychological wellbeing. Early attachment relationships foster integration through attuned, contingent regulation that shape brain development, affect regulation, and stress-response systems. When caregiving is frightening, inconsistent, or marked by non-influence, integrative processes are disrupted. This contributes to the fragmented organisation characteristic of cumulative relational trauma. In psychotherapy, IPNB highlights the therapist's attuned presence as a relational context in which fragmented self--states can be reorganised through co-regulation and reflective engagement.
Intersubjectivity	The relational space between persons in which subjectivity is formed, recognised, and transformed. Intersubjectivity refers to the ongoing, reciprocal processes of affective attunement, misattunement, regulation, and repair through which experience acquires meaning. In this volume, intersubjectivity is understood as foundational to development and therapeutic change, rather than as a secondary exchange between pre-existing, fully formed subjects. See also subjectivity.
Intrapsychic	Refers to the internal organisation of mental life – representations, affects, and defensive processes operating within the individual. In this volume, the intrapsychic is understood as emergent from intersubjective experience, following Benjamin's view that internal structures reflect internalised relational patterns rather than isolated mental events. Intrapsychic organisation remains dynamically linked to the intersubjective field, shaping and being shaped by ongoing relational engagement.
Marked mirroring	The caregiver's reflection of the infant's emotional state in an exaggerated or modified form that signals, implicitly, "this is your feeling, not mine". Marked mirroring supports emotional recognition, differentiation, and regulation.

Mentalisation	The capacity to understand one's own and others' behaviour in terms of underlying mental states such as feelings, intentions, desires, and beliefs. Developed within early attachment relationships and shaped across the lifespan, mentalisation supports emotional regulation, perspective-taking, and flexible relating. In contemporary clinical usage, the concept is most closely associated with the work of Peter Fonagy and colleagues, who emphasise both its centrality to resilience and its variability. Mentalisation operates along a continuum and can collapse under conditions of high arousal or trauma, giving way to more rigid, reactive, or non-mentalising modes of understanding.
Mirror neuron system	Neural circuitry that activates both when an individual performs an action or experiences an emotion and when observing another person perform that action or display that emotion. Thought to underpin empathy and social understanding.
Misattunement	Failures of the caregiver to accurately perceive, respond to, or repair the infant's emotional signals and needs. When chronic or unaddressed, misattunement becomes a significant source of cumulative trauma.
Moment of meeting	An authentic, improvised relational response to a "now moment" in which both participants move beyond prescribed roles to meet each other more fully. In the Boston Change Process Study Group's framework, moments of meeting facilitate change in implicit relational knowing and establish new procedural patterns through shared present experience rather than interpretation.
Motivational systems	In Lichtenberg and Liotti's frameworks, distinct innate systems (e.g., attachment, caregiving, exploration, sexuality) that organise behaviour and experience. Relational disturbance may arise when motivational systems conflict – for example, when attachment needs simultaneously activate expectations of danger or rejection.

Mutual influence	The bidirectional, conscious and unconscious impact that therapist and patient exert on one another. Mutual influence reflects the intersubjective nature of therapeutic work and underscores the inevitability of enactments within the relational field.
Neural plasticity	The nervous system's capacity to reorganise its structure, connectivity, and functional patterns across the lifespan in ways that register developmental, environmental, and relational experience, enabling adaptation and the reworking of embodied patterns within clinical encounters.
Neurobiology	The study of the structure, development, and functioning of the nervous system. In this chapter, the term refers specifically to how early relational experiences shape brain development, affect regulation, and stress-response systems.
Non-influence	The child's repeated experience that their emotional signals, needs, or protests fail to alter the caregiver's response. Over time, experiences of non-influence contribute to the development of cumulative relational trauma, shaping procedural expectations of futility, withdrawal, hyperactivation, or enactment.
Now moment	A moment of heightened affective engagement between patient and therapist that emerges spontaneously and opens possibilities for relational transformation. Distinguished from ordinary interaction by its intensity, unpredictability, and potential to shift implicit relational knowing. When met with authentic engagement, a now moment can become a "moment of meeting" that alters the relational field.
Parental reflective functioning	The caregiver's capacity to consider and reflect upon the child's mental states (thoughts, feelings, intentions) and their own mental states as they pertain to the parent–child relationship. Strongly predictive of secure attachment.

Parentified child	A developmental role-reversal in which the child assumes caregiving or emotional-regulatory functions that belong to the parent. Parentification disrupts relational asymmetry and, when chronic or unacknowledged, becomes a pathway into cumulative relational trauma, placing sustained demands on the child's affective and behavioural capacities. These experiences are procedurally encoded, shaping later expectations of over--responsibility, vigilance, and self-effacement in relationships, including within the therapeutic dyad.
Phenomenological experience	The lived, felt, and relationally organised experience of the individual, encompassing the emotional atmosphere, bodily states, perceptions of others, and the meaning-laden way the world is encountered from the inside. Phenomenological experience refers not merely to what a person feels, but to how their relational environment is subjectively structured, anticipated, and inhabited. See also subjectivity. Whereas subjectivity refers to the emergent organisation of feeling, perception, and meaning shaped within early attachment relationships, phenomenological experience highlights how these internal organisations structure the lived, relational world as it is felt and inhabited.
Polyvagal theory	A neurobiological framework proposed by Stephen Porges, describing how the autonomic nervous system regulates states of social engagement, mobilisation (fight/flight), and immobilisation (shutdown) via the vagus nerve. Emphasises the role of co-regulation within attachment relationships.

Prefrontal cortex (PFC)	A set of cortical regions involved in executive functioning, reflective thought, affect regulation, and the integration of implicit and explicit experience. The prefrontal cortex supports mentalisation, flexible attention, impulse modulation, and the capacity to hold multiple perspectives in mind. Its development is profoundly shaped by early attachment relationships – repeated experiences of co-regulation, marked mirroring, and reliable repair scaffold the maturation of prefrontal networks. Cumulative relational trauma – marked by chronic misattunement, non-influence, or frightening caregiving – can disrupt prefrontal development, leading to difficulties in regulating arousal, symbolising affect, and maintaining reflective stance under stress. When arousal exceeds the window of tolerable affect, prefrontal functioning may collapse, giving way to procedural, survival-based modes of relating. In psychotherapy, the therapist's regulated presence and capacity for informed uncertainty help re-engage prefrontal processes, supporting the gradual integration of dissociated experience and the emergence of more flexible relational organisation.
Preoccupied attachment	An Adult Attachment Interview classification characterised by excessive, confused, or angry preoccupation with attachment relationships. Discourse is often incoherent, with unfinished sentences, tangential associations, and difficulty maintaining narrative focus. The adult equivalent of infant ambivalent-resistant attachment, reflecting hyper-activation of the attachment system and under-regulated emotional expression.
Primal repression	In psychoanalytic theory, an early, pre-verbal form of repression rendering intense archaic experiences inaccessible to consciousness. Conceptually related to implicit memory encoding in infancy.
Procedural expectation	Nonconscious anticipations about how interactions will unfold, based on encoded patterns from previous relational experience. Procedural expectations shape behaviour, affect, and relational engagement without conscious awareness and are revealed through enactments in current relationships, including the therapeutic relationship.

Procedural memory	A form of implicit memory for learned patterns of action, interaction, and relating. Nonconscious in nature and expressed through behaviour rather than verbal recall.
Procedural transformation	A mode of therapeutic change in which implicitly encoded relational patterns are reorganised through lived experience rather than insight. Transformation occurs through "moments of meeting" that transform affective expectations at a sub-symbolic level, gradually developing new relational procedures through the medium of the therapeutic relationship.
Protective shield	Originally Freud's term for the ego's defence against overwhelming stimulation. Reformulated by Khan and Winnicott to describe the caregiver's function in mediating the infant's experience of the external world, protecting against premature impingement. Failure of this protective function contributes to cumulative trauma.
Reflective functioning	A research-based operationalisation of mentalisation, most commonly assessed through the Adult Attachment Interview. Measures the capacity to reflect on mental states in oneself and others.
Relational asymmetry	The inherent imbalance of responsibility and power within caregiving and therapeutic relationships, in which the adult or therapist bears primary responsibility for regulation, containment, and ethical maintenance of the frame.
Relational field	The dynamic, co-created psychological space that emerges between individuals, encompassing affective exchange, implicit expectations, mutual influence, and the organisation of interaction. The relational field is not reducible to either participant; it reflects the ongoing interplay of their histories, self-states, and procedural patterns. In cumulative relational trauma, the field may become shaped by fear, non-influence, or hypervigilance. In psychotherapy, attending to the relational field allows dissociated or enacted material to be recognised, symbolised, and reorganised within the intersubjective space.

Relational neuroscience	An interdisciplinary approach examining how brain development and functioning are shaped within ongoing relational contexts, particularly early caregiving relationships. Emphasises co-regulation, affective attunement, and the embodied nature of interpersonal experience.
Relational template	An implicitly encoded organisational pattern of expectation, affect regulation, and role anticipation formed through repeated early relational experience. Relational templates operate procedurally and are enacted in later relationships, including within the therapeutic dyad.
Relational third	The co-created intersubjective field that exceeds either participant and becomes the locus where dissociated trauma, unmetabolised affect, and new relational possibilities emerge. In a relational-neurodevelopmental frame, the Third functions as the container in which unmentalised experience can be enacted, recognised, and reorganised.
Relational–neurodevelopmental framework	An integrative perspective that understands mind and brain development as emerging from the continuous interplay between relational experience and neurobiological processes. It highlights how interpersonal regulation, affective exchange, and cultural context shape neural organisation, self--development, and patterns of relating across the lifespan.
Repair	The caregiver's efforts to restore emotional connection and attunement following a relational disruption or misattunement. Timely and adequate repair is essential for healthy emotional development and secure attachment.
Representation	The mental organisation of experience in forms that can be held in mind, anticipated, and reflected upon. In psychoanalytic and developmental contexts, representations refer to internalised patterns of expectation about self and others, formed through repeated relational experience. Representations may exist at implicit (procedural) levels or become symbolically elaborated within explicit memory and reflective thought.

Right hemisphere/left hemisphere	In affective neuroscience, the right hemisphere is associated with nonverbal, holistic, and emotionally-charged processing, particularly in early development. The left hemisphere is associated with linear, verbal, and analytical processing. Early attachment experiences particularly shape right-hemisphere development. Therapeutic work involves facilitating integration between implicit (right-hemisphere) and explicit (left-hemisphere) systems.
Role-responsiveness	The therapist's unconscious tendency to occupy roles evoked by the patient's internal relational templates. Roles may reflect dissociated self-states or traumatic relational patterns.
Rupture and repair	The inevitable cycle of misattunement followed by reconnection within caregiving and therapeutic relationships. Successful repair teaches that disruptions can be tolerated and relationships restored.
Screen memories	A psychoanalytic concept referring to memories that are consciously accessible but serve to obscure or "screen" more emotionally charged or traumatic experiences. Such memories often carry symbolic significance rather than historical accuracy.
Second-order representational models	Mental models that represent and reflect upon primary implicit relational patterns, making them available for conscious consideration and potential revision. Created through therapeutic work that brings implicit procedural knowledge into explicit, symbolised awareness.
Secure attachment	An attachment pattern in which the infant uses the caregiver as a secure base for exploration, shows distress during separation, and is readily soothed upon reunion. Associated with consistent, sensitive caregiving.
Secure base	The caregiver's function of providing a reliable foundation of safety from which the child can explore the environment, returning for comfort and reassurance as needed.

Self-state	A relatively discrete, organised pattern of self-experience, affects, and relational expectations that can shift depending on context and activated relational models. Emphasises the multiplicity and context-dependence of self-experience rather than a unified, continuous self-structure.
Sensitive responsiveness	The caregiver's ability to accurately perceive the child's signals and respond promptly and appropriately. Considered the strongest predictor of secure attachment.
Social biofeedback theory	Gergely and Watson's model proposing that the caregiver's marked, contingent mirroring of the infant's emotional expressions functions as feedback, enabling the infant to recognise and regulate affective states.
Social constructivism	An epistemological stance holding that meanings, identities, and relational expectations are formed through social, cultural, and interpersonal processes. Within this volume, social constructivism highlights that what is perceived, and how it is understood, depends on shared narratives and relational contexts. Observation is thus inherently situated and co-constructed rather than neutral or detached.
Somatisation	The expression of psychological distress through bodily symptoms, particularly when emotional experience cannot yet be symbolised or mentalised. From a relational perspective, somatisation is understood as an embodied form of communication rather than merely a symptom to be eliminated.
Still face paradigm	An experimental procedure (Tronick) in which a caregiver maintains an unresponsive expression towards their infant following normal interaction. Demonstrates infants' sensitivity to disruptions in attunement and the importance of timely repair following relational ruptures.
Strange situation procedure (SSP)	A laboratory-based assessment designed to activate the infant's attachment system through brief separations and reunions with the caregiver in the presence of a stranger. Used to classify infant attachment patterns.

Stress-response systems Neurobiological networks that register and respond to perceived threat or challenge, coordinating physiological, emotional, and behavioural responses. These systems develop within caregiving relationships and, when chronically activated, can contribute to cumulative trauma and intergenerational transmission of stress sensitivity.

Subjectivity The lived, embodied, and affective experience of being a person, emerging and shaped developmentally through early relational interactions. Subjectivity is not understood here as a purely intrapsychic or reflective phenomenon, but as an emergent organisation of feeling, perception, and meaning that arises within attachment relationships and is structured by implicit relational experience. It is expressed as much in bodily states, affect regulation, and relational patterns as in conscious thought or narrative. See also Intersubjectivity.

Symbolic representation The capacity to encode experience in language, imagery, or other symbolic forms that allow reflection, communication, and narrative organisation. Symbolic representation depends on the maturation of explicit memory systems and develops within relational contexts that support affect regulation and meaning-making. Disruptions in early relational experience may limit the integration of implicit relational memory into symbolic form, contributing to enactment, dissociation, or difficulties in reflective functioning.

Symbolisation The developmental process through which raw sensory, affective, and relational experience becomes represented in language, imagery, gesture, or thought. Symbolisation enables reflection, communication, and meaning-making, transforming implicit experience into forms that can be mentally held and shared. It depends on early experiences of attuned mirroring and containment. In cumulative relational trauma, symbolisation may be compromised, leaving affective states unformulated or enacted. Psychotherapy provides a relational environment in which previously unsymbolised experience can be named, held, and integrated.

Systems theory (in attachment theory)	A framework for understanding behaviour and development as emerging from dynamic, self-organising interactions within an open system. Bowlby applied systems theory to conceptualise the attachment behavioural system as an organised, context-sensitive system integrating internal states, environmental conditions, and relational cues. This perspective situates attachment within a relational, developmental process rather than a linear, drive-based model.
Therapeutic frame	The set of ethical, temporal, and relational boundaries that provide safety, containment, and predictability. The frame supports attachment security and enables the symbolic elaboration of dissociated or unrepresented experience.
Transference	The largely unconscious activation, within current relationships, of expectations, affects, and relational patterns shaped by earlier significant relationships. In contemporary relational psychoanalysis, transference is understood as co-constructed and enacted within the therapeutic relationship rather than as a distortion originating solely within the patient. From an attachment perspective, transference reflects the activation of internal working models and procedural memory in present relationships.
Transmission gap	The observation that parental sensitivity alone does not fully explain how adult attachment states of mind predict infant attachment patterns. Parental reflective functioning helps to narrow this gap.
Traumatic transference/traumatic countertransference	A relational configuration in which dissociated traumatic experience is reactivated within the therapeutic dyad.

Triangulation	The developmental process through which the child moves from an early two-person, symbiotic organisation with the primary caregiver into a three-person relational field. The introduction of a third – traditionally the father, but functionally any figure or force that disrupts the closed dyad – creates space for separation, difference, and the recognition of the caregiver's independent subjectivity. Triangulation supports the emergence of symbolic thought, perspective-taking, and the capacity to negotiate complex relational configurations. When the triangulating function is absent or compromised, the dyad may remain insufficiently differentiated, contributing to difficulties with individuation, boundary formation, and the toleration of relational complexity in later life.
Unmentalised experience	Affective or relational material that has not yet been symbolised or integrated into reflective functioning. Such experience often emerges through enactment, bodily communication, or dissociated self-states.
Unresolved attachment	An Adult Attachment Interview classification indicating unresolved trauma or loss, characterised by lapses in discourse coherence when discussing traumatic experiences. Strongly predictive of disorganised attachment in offspring.
Vagus nerve/polyvagal theory	The autonomic pathway central to regulation and social engagement. Polyvagal Theory highlights the ventral vagal system as the neurobiological substrate of co-regulation. In clinical practice, the therapist's regulated physiology becomes a biological bridge that helps the patient shift from defensive states toward safety and receptivity.
Vitality affects	Daniel Stern's term for dynamic, kinetic qualities of experience (e.g., surging, fading, explosive, gentle) that characterise the felt sense of being alive. Distinguished from categorical emotions (happy, sad, angry), vitality affects describe the temporal, intensive, and textural dimensions of experience and are communicated through rhythm, timing, and intensity in early interactions.

Window of tolerable affect	The range of emotional intensity an individual can experience and process without becoming overwhelmed, dissociating, or shutting down; the zone in which affect is accessible, meaningful, and can be worked with therapeutically.

Index

For Product Safety Concerns and Information please contact our EU
representative GPSR@taylorandfrancis.com
Taylor & Francis Verlag GmbH, Kaufingerstraße 24, 80331 München, Germany

www.ingramcontent.com/pod-product-compliance
Ingram Content Group UK Ltd.
Pitfield, Milton Keynes, MK11 3LW, UK
UKHW022021180926
475701UK00005B/970

* 9 7 8 1 0 4 1 3 3 4 7 8 1 *